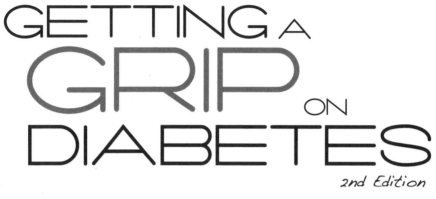

# GETTING A GRIP ON DIABETES

2nd Edition

## QUICK TIPS & TECHNIQUES FOR KIDS & TEENS

*Spike and Bo Loy*

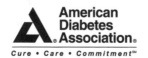

**American Diabetes Association®**

*Cure • Care • Commitment*℠

*Director, Book Publishing,* John Fedor; *Managing Editor, Book Publishing,* Abe Ogden; *Acquisitions Editor, Consumer Books,* Robert Anthony; *Editor,* Rebecca Lanning; *Production Manager,* Melissa Sprott; *Composition,* ADA; *Cover Design,* Pixiedesign; *Printer,* Worzalla Printing.

Printed in the United States of America
1 3 5 7 9 10 8 6 4 2

The suggestions and information contained in this publication are generally consistent with the Clinical Practice Recommendations and other policies of the American Diabetes Association, but they do not represent the policy or position of the Association or any of its boards or committees. Reasonable steps have been taken to ensure the accuracy of the information presented. However, the American Diabetes Association cannot ensure the safety or efficacy of any product or service described in this publication. Individuals are advised to consult a physician or other appropriate health care professional before undertaking any diet or exercise program or taking any medication referred to in this publication. Professionals must use and apply their own professional judgment, experience, and training and should not rely solely on the information contained in this publication before prescribing any diet, exercise, or medication. The American Diabetes Association—its officers, directors, employees, volunteers, and members—assumes no responsibility or liability for personal or other injury, loss, or damage that may result from the suggestions or information in this publication.

♾ The paper in this publication meets the requirements of the ANSI Standard Z39.48-1992 (permanence of paper).

ADA titles may be purchased for business or promotional use or for special sales. To purchase more than 50 copies of this book at a discount, or for custom editions of this book with your logo, contact Lee Romano Sequeira, Special Sales & Promotions, at the address below, or at LRomano@diabetes.org or 703-299-2046.

For all other inquiries, please call 1-800-DIABETES.

American Diabetes Association
1701 North Beauregard Street
Alexandria, Virginia 22311

**Library of Congress Cataloging-in-Publication Data**

Loy, Spike Nasmyth, 1980–
  Getting a grip on diabetes : quick tips and techniques for kids and teens / Spike Nasmyth Loy and Bo Nasmyth Loy. — 2nd ed.
    p. cm.
  Includes index.
  ISBN-13: 978-1-58040-255-2 (alk. paper)
  1. Diabetes in children—Juvenile literature. 2. Diabetes in children—Patients—Home care—Juvenile literature. 3. Diabetes in adolescence—Patients—Home care—Juvenile literature. [1. Diabetes. 2. Diseases.] I. Loy, Bo Nasmyth, 1982– . II. Title.
  RJ420.D5L695 2007
  618.92'462—dc22
                          2006100208

# Contents

# Foreword

Until the publication of *Getting a Grip on Diabetes* in 2000, I had seen nothing with which a young patient could directly identify. This new second edition shares diabetes know-how through childhood, the teen years, and college. The obvious success of Spike and Bo in dealing with their diabetes will inspire other young people.

After almost fifty years of practicing medicine, I can look back on significant experience in treating pediatric patients with diabetes. When the diagnosis of diabetes is first made, families are presented with extensive information on diabetes management and how to balance insulin, food, and exercise. What is frequently missing is the patient's point of view. With the publication of the first edition of *Getting a Grip on Diabetes*, I was struck by the accessibility of Spike and Bo's firsthand experience and their easy style in communicating with their peers. Their stories enable my patients to turn dealing with diabetes into a shared adventure.

Spike and Bo were first diagnosed with type 1 diabetes (at seven and six years of age, respectively). Now, more than fifteen years later, their accomplishments are staggering. In addition to their spectacular academic and athletic success, their efforts to promote awareness and education about type 1 diabetes have received community and national accolades.

As Spike and Bo have grown to adulthood and adapted to life on the pump, the audience for this book will also grow. It has become a volume that young adults, as well as kids and teens, can relate to and be helped by. I wholeheartedly recommend *Getting a Grip on Diabetes* to young people and their families. No family dealing with diabetes should be without this book.

MARTIN E. BERGER, M.D.

# Acknowledgments

We thank everyone who contributed time and energy to making this book and especially all our friends who have helped us deal with diabetes all along the way. Thanks to our awesome neighbors for learning how to take care of us: the Wildes, the Clems, the MacDonalds, the Sakamotos, the Boccalis, the Amestoys, and the whole of Upper Ojai. Thanks to Kevin and Erik and the boys for making sure we ate and for paddling us out of the water and to the guys up at school for the frosting treatment. Thanks to all of our teachers, coaches, and school administrators for taking care of kids with diabetes at school and for assigning the homework that became this book.

Thanks to the kids and parents from Kids with Diabetes, Inc., for their priceless input and feedback and their perspectives. We especially thank Patty Conlan for her compassion and her work with both the book and the group.

Thanks to Dr. Marty Berger and Aunt Gebo for editing, input, and especially for putting up with all the phone calls when we had late-night questions. Thanks to Grandma Virginia for reviewing the manuscript and for putting up the big bucks so we could continue giving away copies. Thanks to Shed and June Behar and David and Jana Hedman for all their input and assistance. A special thanks to Herman Rush for his guidance and for helping bring our ideas to fruition.

Thanks also to Timothy Teague, Larry Hagman, and Gloria Forgea for their contributions and support. Big thanks go to Sherrye Landrum at the ADA for treating us well and taking an interest in seeing this project through. We thank our congressman, Elton Gallegly, for his unswerving support both at home and in Washington. Thanks to Ken Pitzer and Cygnus for hiring Spike and for their progress with the Glucowatch. Thank you to Medtronic MiniMed, not only for being so supportive of our books and helping with our diabetes management, but also for hiring Bo and for all the miracles you perform each day for everyone living with diabetes.

Since the first edition of *Getting a Grip* came out, we've received truckloads of input from kids with diabetes and grownups who care. We want to especially thank Julia Halprin Jackson, Mary Costello Wright, and Derrick Crowe for their contributions. Also, since the first printing we've been involved in some very exciting research work here in California. We owe a huge thanks to Robert Klein for envisioning, tirelessly promoting, and passing Proposition 71, the Stem Cell Initiative. Thanks to everyone at the California Institute for Stem Cell Research and all the people who helped Bob create it—Governor Arnold Schwarzenegger, California State Senator Deborah Ortiz, and the folks at Americans for Cures.

A big thank you goes to doctors Kevin Kaiserman and Rocky Wilson for their tireless contributions to Camp Conrad-Chinnock and for contributing to this book.

We want to thank Dr. Ronald Chochinov for his many contributions and for his tireless work for kids with diabetes. Thank you to the wonderful Debbie Warner for teaching so many kids how to go on the pump, including us, and for always being there when we need her.

Thank you to Marc Weigensberg, MD, for his insight, research, and support and for his dedication to everyone with diabetes.

We also thank everyone who worked with us on research at our ranch—long before we wrote this book. So, thanks to Dr. Patrick Soon Shiong for getting us involved with and excited about islet cell research in the first place. Huge thanks to Cobby Oxford, Ray Edwards, Gayle Mortenson from the Pig Improvement Company, Dave Ochletree, John Perry, Phil Schmit, Jake Colborn, Chris and Gan Nash, Margaret Stangeland, and Mandy and Wes MacDonald for all of their work with the pigs and the research; it truly was a community effort, and you'll never know how much it meant to two kids with diabetes to see all of their neighbors coming together and helping us.

Finally, we want to thank our family—Dad and our sisters, Jen and Mary, for all of their work and input on this book, and especially Mom for her editing, publishing, organizing, and work as our unofficial agent. But far more important, we thank them for their love and devotion and for always making sure we were all right. We love you.

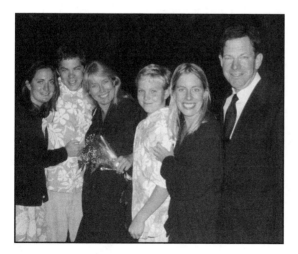

The Loy family at Mom's college graduation.

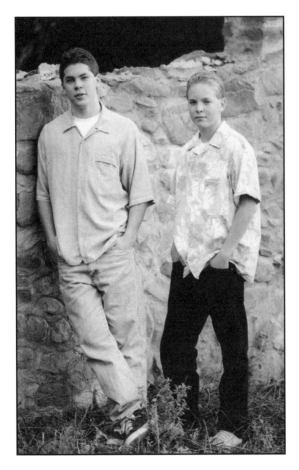

**Spike and Bo in front of the Castle.**

# Introduction

Spike Loy was diagnosed with type 1 diabetes at age seven. Bo Loy was diagnosed at age six. Spike and Bo are brothers who grew up on a forty-acre ranch in rural Upper Ojai, California, with their parents and their sisters, Jenny and Mary.

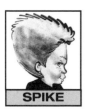

In his senior year at Nordhoff High School, Spike was valedictorian, homecoming king, ASB Vice President, and a National Merit Scholar. He has been to Ecuador and the Galapagos Islands, Costa Rica, South Africa, and Swaziland, among other countries.

Spike recently graduated from Stanford University with a degree in human biology and plans to work in the field of diabetes law. As Spike says, "I am interested in this field because on Thanksgiving Day of 1987, I was diagnosed with insulin-dependent diabetes. Exactly one year later, on Thanksgiving Day of 1988, my six-year-old brother Bo was diagnosed with insulin-dependent diabetes."

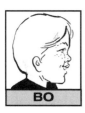

Bo graduated from Nordhoff High School in 2000, where he too excelled academically, athletically, and socially. He had a 4.3 grade point average and was the ASB Vice President. He was on the honor roll, served in leadership positions, worked as an associate editor on the school newspaper, and played varsity soccer. Bo recently graduated, magna cum laude, from the University of Southern California with a major in biomedical engineering and a minor in philosophy. Along with his brother, he has had many adventures around the world, including surfing in Costa Rica, backpacking in Yosemite, and trekking in the South African veldt. Bo is an avid surfer and snowboarder. He plays racquetball and enjoys USC football.

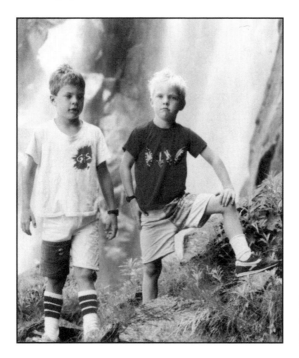

**Spike and Bo striking a pose in Yosemite.**

Bo says, "You can do anything when you have diabetes. Spike and I have years of experience dealing with diabetes. We think our experience will help you, and this book will make your life easier. Toward the end of the 1997–98 school year, we began putting down our thoughts about dealing with diabetes. Soon we realized how much we have learned over the years through trial and error. We began sharing this information with other kids, and so this book was born. *Getting a Grip* is meant to help kids with diabetes, their families, and their friends. When you have diabetes, you need to develop a support group. This book will show you how. *Getting a Grip on Diabetes* is about what you can do!"

## YOU CAN DO ANYTHING!

People with diabetes can do everything that anyone else can do. You just have to understand your diabetes and learn about the things you need to do to make your life run smoothly. You will have to be a little more careful about eating and exercising than your friends. Inside this book are tips and tricks about how to get along at school, what to do when you're playing sports, what to do when you're feeling a low blood sugar, how to handle traveling around the globe and how to pack the extra supplies that will make your trip a breeze, and more.

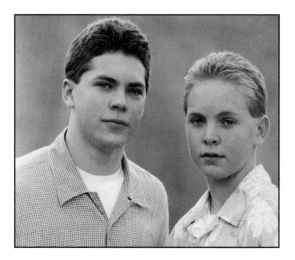

**Spike and Bo as newly published authors.**

In the back of the book, you will find documents that we encourage you to reproduce and give to the people you know. We have found that once your friends and their parents, your teachers, and your coaches have an understanding of what diabetes is and the special needs that come along with it, they will be eager to help.

## *GETTING A GRIP*—UPDATED

A lot has happened in the lives of both Bo and Spike since first publishing *Getting a Grip* back in 2000. After graduating with a double major from USC, Bo traveled to China, Ireland, and Spain, got a job as a consultant, and now lives and surfs in Manhattan Beach, California. He plans to work for a few years before possibly going back to business school and someday running a biotech company, working to improve the lives of kids with diabetes and eventually curing it.

Spike graduated from college, got married, and has headed off to Columbia Law School in New York City, far away from home on the East Coast. Spike decided against medical research after he realized his strengths would be put to better use in a courtroom than in a laboratory. (Bo could have told you this long ago: "He likes to argue!") Bo thinks Spike's first chemistry grades may have had something to do with it, too. Spike is planning to study health law and dreams of one day working for the California Institute of Regenerative Medicine (the new $3 billion stem cell institute in California), helping fight for a cure for diabetes.

A lot has also happened in the world of diabetes since 2000. Insulin pumps have improved dramatically and now come with all sorts of new bells and whistles. Both of us have been on insulin pumps since December 2002; our numbers are even better than they used to be, and dealing with diabetes has gotten even easier. New insulins have been developed that act more naturally and help simplify our lives. Blood test meters have gotten smaller and smaller and now require so little blood Bo can't even feel his tests (which, by the way, he doesn't do on his fingers anymore—now he tests on his arm). The future looks even better, with the development of continuous monitors that will be able to test your blood sugar automatically all day long and "closed loop" systems that will someday soon monitor blood sugars and deliver insulin automatically. Stem cell research is very new, but the possibility of replacing islet cells in the pancreas is super exciting. Scientists are working on this research as we write this.

With all the new things happening in our lives and in the diabetes world, we thought it was high time to update *Getting a Grip*. As we've gotten older and wiser (at least we've gotten older), we've discovered new techniques that help make diabetes even easier to deal with. We still share new diabetes adventures with each other in case a situation arises for Spike that Bo just went through (see Bo's story about his pump malfunctioning on the biggest football day of his life). We hope these stories will make it a little easier for you to handle new situations and adventures, too.

## WHAT THE DOC SAYS:

Marc J. Weigensberg, MD, Director of Pediatric Endocrinology at Los Angeles County University of Southern California Medical Center, has contributed to the "What the Doc Says" sections of this book. Dr. Weigensberg is Associate Professor of Clinical Pediatrics at the Keck USC School of Medicine, where he is currently developing innovative interventions utilizing mind-body modalities designed to prevent type 2 diabetes in overweight youth.

# 1 What Is Diabetes?

One of the little-known organs in your body is the pancreas. Inside it are cells called islet (pronounced eye-let) cells. Islet cells produce insulin in most people's bodies, but when you have diabetes, they don't. Insulin is like a key that fits into the doors to the cells in your body, unlocks them, and lets sugar (glucose) get into them. If your body doesn't make any insulin "keys," all the doors on most of your body's cells stay locked, and glucose can't get to where it is supposed to go. When this happens, the sugar builds up in your blood, leading to high blood sugar levels, while at the same time, your cells are starving. All the food and drink you consume just passes through your system. This is why you have to pee a lot, and you get dehydrated.

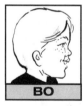

BO

When your pancreas works as it should, it releases just the right amount of insulin every time you eat. The insulin takes your food to the cells, leaving a backup supply of sugar in the blood. In kids with diabetes, this doesn't work, so we use a pump or "shoot up" (inject) insulin. Since we put insulin into our bodies at certain times, it goes to work at certain times, no matter what we eat. If we inject a lot of insulin but we don't eat any food, the insulin takes all the sugar to our cells at once. There is very little sugar left in the bloodstream, so we get low blood sugar (hypoglycemia). If we don't take any insulin and we eat, our bodies have no insulin. The cells can't get the sugar, so it just builds up in our blood, and we get high blood sugar (hyperglycemia).

## WHAT THE DOC SAYS:

The type of diabetes that many children and teenagers get is type 1 diabetes, which occurs when the insulin-producing beta cells (a type of islet cell) in the pancreas have been destroyed by the body's immune system. Usually, the immune system fights viruses and bacteria and attacks foreign substances. However, in the case of diabetes, these antibodies attack the beta cells and destroy them. The only way for the body to get the insulin that it needs is from an injection with a syringe or from an insulin pump.

**Why Do We Shoot Up Insulin Instead of Getting a New Pancreas?** Because the risk of getting an organ transplant is higher than the benefits. Getting a new organ requires surgery, and that can be dangerous. The new islet cell transplants that you hear about in the news are simpler and safer to do, but when you put someone else's body parts into your own, you have to take lots of serious drugs to keep those body parts safe and healthy. The body tries to reject them. Pumping or taking daily injections of insulin is actually the safest solution to controlling diabetes right now.

**How Did We Develop Diabetes?** One of the leading theories is that, for some reason, our immune system attacked and destroyed our islet cells. Our white blood cells, which usually attack bacteria and viruses in our bodies, thought that our islet cells looked like viruses and killed them. For this reason, we can't just take injections of new islet cells either. Our white blood cells are programmed to think that anything that looks like an islet cell is an enemy, so they attack even new ones.

**WHAT THE DOC SAYS:**

The only "cure" for type 1 diabetes that we have right now is a pancreas transplant. However, people who get this transplant have to take strong drugs to suppress their immune system for the rest of their lives, which puts them at risk for infection and some types of cancer. It is not an easy choice to make. Pancreas transplants are not usually done in children. Islet cell transplants, which are currently being studied, are easier to do, but they are not yet available for children either.

Our family spent many years helping with research involving transplanting islet cells into people's bodies. Scientists are working to replace the islet cells we used to have and to protect them from our immune systems with little "bubble" shields. Transplanted islet cells will work just like the ones we had before diabetes. The bubbles protect the islet cells from white blood cells that would attack them. The porous bubbles allow sugar to enter, which stimulates the new islets to make insulin. The insulin can then flow out of the bubble into the bloodstream, while the bubble keeps the white blood cells out and the islet cells alive. We hope that research like this will soon make books like ours obsolete.

## HOW DO YOU KNOW WHEN YOU'RE LOW?

If your blood sugar is lower than 80 mg/dl, you might start to feel low. This feeling is caused by low blood sugar; you feel down, and you have less energy. Once it is below 60 mg/dl, you probably will feel it. Most people feel low blood sugars, but not everybody does. Whether or not you feel a low blood sugar has to do with the rate of change. If your blood sugar drops rapidly, you're more likely to feel it. If it's dropping gradually, you might miss it. (Since we usually feel it, we are writing from our experience.) As your sugar drops down to around 30 mg/dl, you start feeling quite bad. Sometimes you can mistake high blood sugar feelings for low blood sugar and vice versa.

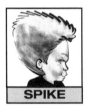

The best thing to do when you are feeling a little out of it is first to drink or eat something and then test your sugar. If you are really low, the few minutes you spend checking your sugar can be when you pass out, so drinking or eating right away is your best bet. If you are high, well, you will be a little higher after eating, but it's better to be safe than sorry. When you are low, you may experience these symptoms:

* **Headache:** This is usually my first sign of low blood sugar—and Bo's, too. You may also feel rather lightheaded or a little dizzy. (Headaches are often associated with high sugars as well.)
* **Stomach ache:** If your stomach feels either knotted up or very empty, chances are that you're low. My stomach usually feels empty when I am around 50–60 mg/dl and gets a severely tight feeling when I am closer to 40 mg/dl.
* **Shakiness:** If you think you might be low, try holding your hand straight and steady in front of your face. If it is shaking pretty uncontrollably, then you can bet that you are low. The shakier it is, the lower you are. If you don't even feel like you can hold your hand up, then you know you are low and should drink something like fruit juice or milk right away.

* **Crying, violently upset:** If you get extremely unreasonable and unruly, you may be low. Of course, you might just be mad, but if it is first thing in the morning and you get irritable at someone for no good reason, you may be experiencing extremely low blood sugar. However, at this point you probably won't listen to reason, and you may be convinced that you are just plain pissed and won't believe that you are having blood sugar problems. Test your blood and see. After having my mom show me that I was desperately low when I was acting up, I began to believe her. Now I realize that you can't make a rational thought when you're low.

There are other signs of more drastic lows, but usually you will not be able to notice them. These include passing out or fainting, not waking up, walking around but not responding, and, at the worst, convulsions. I have never experienced convulsions, but one morning Bo had one. He wouldn't get out of bed—no matter what—so we finally yelled at him and put him on the couch, thinking he was just being stubborn. He didn't touch his breakfast either, and again we blamed it on his stubbornness. Then he lay back down and started twitching. We were able to get him back to normal by squirting frosting under his lip and force-feeding him juice and ice cream. It was hard to get him to eat, because when you are low you just don't feel like eating anything and definitely don't feel like listening. We didn't send him to school that day, either. Hopefully, you can recognize the early warning signs of low blood sugar and avoid major problems altogether by eating a little, so you can get on with your life.

Once you get the hang of diabetes, you will recognize lows as they are coming on. Even after ten years, though, you may still have some really big lows. It's OK—no one's perfect. Lows are just part of life.

Your blood sugar level is determined by the balance between what you eat, the insulin you take, how much you exercise, and, to some degree, your emotional state. Everyone with type 1 diabetes will experience low blood sugar (hypoglycemia) at times. If you take care of it right away by eating or drinking some carbohydrate, you can avoid passing out or having convulsions.

Everyone has his or her own unique symptoms of low blood sugar, and you will come to recognize how your own body feels when you're low. Hypoglycemia is somewhat like having your car run out of gas, which then sputters and spits until you fill it again with gas. Your body relies on the fuel of glucose to keep it running, especially your brain, and it will do all it can do to keep glucose flowing to your brain. As your blood sugar drops and you start to run out of fuel, your body secretes glucagon, adrenaline, and other hormones to keep the sugar level up. These lead to the symptoms of shakiness, sweating, and palpitations (heart pounding). If the sugar level continues to drop, you start to experience the symptoms of lack of sugar to the brain, which can include drowsiness, light-headedness, headache, irritability, and hunger.

Pay attention to what your symptoms are. Write them down for your teachers and coaches on the sheet (pages 140–141) that tells them what to do to treat your low blood sugar. When you have any symptoms of low blood sugar, it's time to fuel up (eat)! Take 15 g of carbohydrate (for example, 4 oz of fruit juice, 6 lifesavers, or 3 glucose tablets) and then test your blood sugar. Expect to feel better in 10–15 minutes. If you don't, eat another 15 g of carbohydrate. Remember to always keep boxed fruit juice, hard candies, glucose tablets, or tubes of frosting like the ones that Bo and Spike use with you at all times for those unpredictable lows.

# HOW DO YOU KNOW
# WHEN YOU'RE HIGH?

High blood sugar is having too much sugar in your blood and your brain. High blood sugar levels, 240 mg/dl and above, are not too bad in the short run, but over a long period of time (years), constant high sugar levels lead to complications. Having too much sugar in your blood makes all of your body's filters work overtime, and they may quit early. Don't be scared by a few high sugars. If you find yourself uncontrollably high for over a week or so, contact your doctor. Remember, if you just can't get your sugars to stabilize perfectly, it is always better to run slightly high than too low.

Here are some things you feel or notice when you're high:

* **Thirst:** When your body has too much sugar floating around in it, it needs to balance itself. You get thirsty. It is a good idea to go ahead and drink a lot when this happens. Water is the best thing, but any sugar-free non-carbonated drink will have a good effect. Drinking a lot leads to some of the other symptoms.
* **Need to urinate:** In order to get rid of the sugar, you need to pee frequently. So, if you find yourself having to use the bathroom a couple of times in the same hour, you may want to test your sugar and, if it is high, take some insulin. Safety tip: Never inject insulin without testing your blood sugar!
* **Your pee is clear:** When there is a lot of sugar in your blood, your urine is very light; there's nothing yellow about it. Check your sugar when you have clear urine. If it stays clear for a long time and your sugar is high, do a urine test and check for ketones (see pages 113–114).

* **Clammy:** Bo and I think getting clammy and sweating is just another way your body is trying to regain its balance. My palms often sweat when I have high blood sugar. But sometimes my palms get sweaty when I get real low, too, so always be sure to test when you feel funny.

* **Energy loss:** You might think that with a high blood sugar you would have more energy, but this is not the case. High blood sugar means that a lot of sugar is in your blood and your brain, but it's not in your cells where you need it and you may feel pretty lackluster. When this happens, you will have to increase your dosage of long-lasting insulin (like Lantus) or increase your basal rate (pumpers).

## DO GROWTH SPURTS AFFECT YOUR BLOOD SUGAR?

Often when you are going through growth spurts, your sugars will start to rise. Your normal insulin dose is related to your height and weight. However, when you grow, your body releases hormones that can interfere with insulin action. For this reason, you will often have to increase your dosage by a few units per day. Once the growth spurt is over, though, insulin action will return to normal, and you may experience a few lows because of your increased dosage, but not always. Be ready for this, and carry extra food. Once insulin action returns to normal, bring your dosage slightly back down. You don't have to get an OK from your doctor to change your dosage around just a little. Just make sure the changes make sense and don't put you at risk for hypoglycemia—what we call "crashing." Any large or long-term changes in your insulin dosage should be approved by your doctor, but you don't need to double-check absolutely every time you make a slight change.

High blood sugar (hyperglycemia) can be caused by too much food; by not taking enough insulin; or by anything that places the body under stress, such as physical illness or a lot of emotional stress. When your blood sugar level stays consistently high, your kidneys become overloaded and sugar is then lost in the urine, taking water with it. This makes you urinate a lot. It also makes you thirsty, so you drink a lot as your body tries to make up for the extra water lost in the urine. Many people also report feeling tired, or just "different," and knowing their sugar is high. Feeling "clammy" is more commonly a symptom of low blood sugar, but if it is one of your symptoms of high blood sugar, too, please pay attention to it. A single high blood sugar is not an emergency. But if your high blood sugar won't come down, you may have problems if you also start producing ketones (see pages 113–115). Be careful, and take care of it right away. The treatment is generally to take more insulin and drink lots of water or other sugar-free fluids. If you haven't discussed with your doctor exactly how to adjust your insulin doses when your sugar levels are high, it's better to call and ask for advice than to just guess.

# 2 Getting Organized

## THE KIT

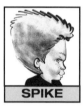

SPIKE

"The Kit" is the name Bo and I use for the carrying case in which I keep all my diabetes products (sometimes I refer to it as "My Life in a Bag"). I carry my kit with me everywhere I go. I take it when I go out to dinner; I take it to school; I take it when I spend the night away from home; I take it in the car every time I drive anywhere. Even if I plan on returning home before my next meal, I bring my kit, because you never know when you'll be stuck on a freeway or the Big One will hit. (We live in California; I'm thinking earthquake.) It is always best to plan for the worst and to be totally prepared. One of the most important points about the kit is to keep it cool. Ice packs work very well. I keep three or four in the freezer at all times, so I can replace the pack every day.

Carry your kit with you everywhere you go. The kit contains an insulin kit (or pump supplies, if you use an insulin pump) and a meter kit:

### Insulin kit
* insulin bottles or insulin pen
* syringes (plenty extra, just in case)
* an injecting device if you use one

## Meter kit

* lancets
* test strips
* a finger or arm pricker
* a glucose monitor and test strips (mine is a Freestyle Tracker)
* frosting or glucose tablets (in case you get really low)
* a granola bar or candy bar
* identification (that says you have diabetes and also lists emergency contacts)
* alcohol swabs to sterilize your finger or arm (optional; Bo and I don't use them)

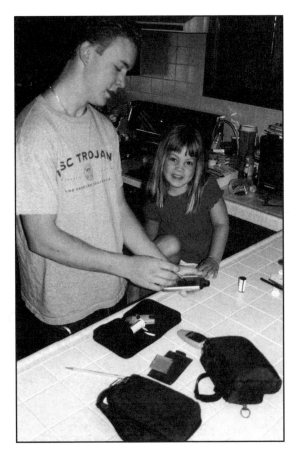

**Bo and Laura discussing meters.**

## Pumpers

\* insulin pump supplies

\* extra infusion sites and reservoirs

\* syringes in case your pump doesn't work

My favorite carrying case is the Medicool Dia-Pak. I can keep my ice pack separate from the insulin bottles, so I don't have to worry about my insulin getting too cold. I keep my blood testing stuff in a "meter" kit bag. I put my insulin kit in the fridge when I'm home, and then both kits go in my carrying case when I go out.

Nowadays, I keep all my blood testing stuff (Freestyle Tracker or strips, lancets, and my pricker) in a separate kit that came with my meter. I just put my whole insulin kit with needles, insulin, ice pack, and all in the fridge when I am hanging out somewhere for a while. I leave it in there overnight and sometimes just leave the ice pack in it in the fridge. I keep my meter kit out of the fridge because meters don't work when they are cold. When I leave the house, I either put my whole meter kit in my insulin kit or strap them together. (Some kits come with a Velcro strap. That can be very useful, but be careful that they don't come undone while you are walking around).

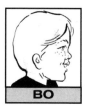
**BO**

Now that we're pumping our kits have evolved. Mine just has my meter, strips, lancets, and frosting in it. It's small enough to fit in my coat pocket!

What a great idea to be this organized every day! The kit is a diabetes care pack that you can take everywhere, and it contains everything you need to treat low blood sugar, such as fruit juice or three glucose tablets. Since these rapid-acting sugar sources only last a short time, it is important to also have a snack with you that acts more slowly but lasts longer, such as granola bars or peanut butter or cheese crackers. Your blood glucose meter and strips are tools to check your blood sugars. If your meter doesn't store your readings, it is helpful to carry a small logbook and pen in your kit so that you can record your blood sugars. This will help you keep track of patterns of sugar levels. For example, you might be able to see that you have low blood sugar every afternoon after soccer practice. This will help you adjust your insulin dose. Instead of syringes and insulin bottles, many people carry insulin pens to make it simpler to take their insulin when they are away from home.

## THE COOLER

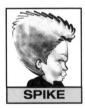

**SPIKE**

The Cooler was my single most important possession throughout elementary school, and it evolved to adapt to my high school life as well. Personally, I think even kids who don't have diabetes would benefit greatly from always having a well-packed cooler on hand. Fortunately for us, we always had an excuse for keeping one. Every morning, I packed my cooler with my snacks in brown paper bags and my special low blood sugar stash and took it to school. It sat under my desk, and every two hours I ate one of my snacks. When I got low, there was always plenty of other stuff in it.

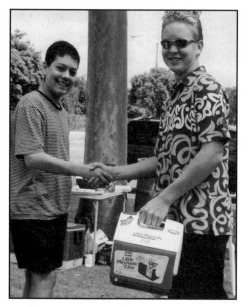

**Bo giving a cooler to a new member of the playgroup.**

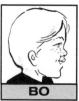
BO

Who is Spike kidding? Mom packed our coolers!

For low blood sugars, my elementary school cooler contained:

* frosting
* Gatorade
* granola bars
* Cheez-Its
* cookies (whatever your favorite kind is)
* jerky
* caramels

I thought I was pretty cool when I got into junior high school, so I no longer wanted to take a Little Igloo cooler to school. A lot of the food items can be transferred to a backpack and a locker, but you shouldn't let your cooler go to waste since it has been with you for so long. I carried the same cooler packed with the same goodies and kept it in my favorite teacher's classroom. That way my food was always nearby, and I didn't have to worry about those mean little seventh and eighth graders making fun of my cooler.

The cooler makes your teachers' lives easier, too. The cooler-in-the-teacher's-class method works best when the cooler also contains a sheet of paper that lists your symptoms of low blood sugar and gives instructions to help you with the situation (see pages 140–141).

Once you have a car, you can put a cooler in there to keep your insulin cool. My car cooler contains:

✳ the same foods listed on page 15
✳ my insulin kit (see pages 11–13)
✳ my extra pump supplies (see pages 92–93)
✳ other medication (I am the only one of my friends who always has Benadryl and Tylenol on hand. This has nothing to do with diabetes, but it sure is handy.)

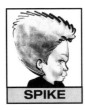

Your cooler equals freedom. Once you get this routine down, you can do anything! Keep a cooler at home, at school, and in each family car. Fill the coolers with frosting, Gatorade, and cookies (we call these "short" foods; see chapter 18); Cheez-Its (a "medium" food); and jerky and peanuts ("long" foods).

SPIKE

> Tape the "Symptoms of Low Blood Sugar" document (pages 140–141) in the top of every cooler. When the symptoms occur (when you are very low), one of your friends will know how to help you.

# THE DIABETES DRAWER

Just as the cooler and the kit are convenient places to keep all of our diabetes supplies when we are away from home, certain kitchen drawers are ideal places for storing things at home. Our diabetes drawer is right under the counter top where we draw our insulin and shoot up.

The diabetes drawer contains:

* needles
* lancets
* alcohol swabs
* finger or arm pricker
* injector
* blood glucose meter kit (meter, strips, lancets, and pricker)
* glucagon kit
* our kits (when not in use, minus the ice pack and the insulin, which go in the refrigerator). Sometimes, though, we put our

whole insulin kit in the fridge; just remember to keep your meter kit out of the fridge.

Insulin needs to be kept cool at all times. When insulin gets too hot, it goes bad. If you are experiencing high sugars, it may be because your insulin is bad due to overheating. Throw it out, and start a new bottle. Sometimes, when you start a new bottle, you may experience lows because the insulin is more potent than the insulin in the old bottle.

### WHAT THE DOC SAYS:

Organization is important for everyone. Once you get organized as Bo and Spike suggest, you have more time to do other things you want to do without wasting time trying to find the supplies that you need when a situation arises or it's time to go to school.

It is true that new insulin is sometimes more potent than old insulin. But if you don't mix your insulin well enough, the active insulin molecules may settle in the bottle and make the end of the vial more potent. Studies show that you need to roll the vial about 20 times to mix the insulin.

## THE FRIDGE: TIPS FOR STORING YOUR SUPPLIES

We use the butter drawer in our refrigerator for storing our insulin. The butter drawer is ideal because it closes. When we forget to close it, our insulin often flies out when we open the door, and sometimes the insulin bottle breaks. Using the butter drawer properly can save money (and the mockery family members enjoy bestowing on you). Use a specific shelf in the freezer door for ice packs. This way you will always know where they are. Every time you come home, unpack your kit and return all insulin to the butter drawer and ice packs to the freezer door shelf. This will ensure that you always have frozen ice packs and potent insulin. Put your meter kit back in the diabetes drawer.

Keep a glucagon kit in your diabetes drawer or in the fridge. Glucagon is like a security blanket. If you are ever drastically low, someone can inject you with glucagon to raise your blood sugar. See pages 119–120 for more about glucagon.

When you're at other people's homes, go ahead and put your insulin kit in their refrigerator. This will keep everything cool, and you won't lose anything. If you can remember to retrieve it, put the ice pack in their freezer, but keeping it with the kit in the fridge will serve your purpose as well. Keep your meter kit in your backpack or cooler.

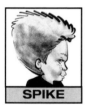

If you have a separate kit for your monitor, or even a pocket in which you can put it, it is best to keep it out of the fridge. If you do throw it in the fridge you will have to wait a few minutes for it to warm up to room temperature before you can test.

Having everything organized and standardized makes my life much easier and eliminates the chance of forgetting to shoot up. You might think that would be hard to forget to do, but once you break your routine (like when summer starts or when you're at a friend's house), you do things in the wrong order. The more systematic your insulin setup is, the less chance there is for error.

# 3 Elementary School

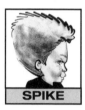

**SPIKE**

I was diagnosed with type 1 diabetes when I was seven years old, just two months after I started the second grade. I made it through elementary school with hardly any diabetes-related problems. The main reason was because my family let every single person at the school (and in the entire town for that matter) know that I had diabetes and informed them what to do if I were to experience low blood sugars.

Here are a few things you and your parents should do:

* **Arrange parent-teacher conferences.** Before school starts, meet with all of the teachers and faculty at the school and instruct them not only on worst-case-scenario procedures but also on the daily needs of a kid with diabetes, such as needing to eat in class and using the restroom frequently when blood sugars are high. You can download a sample diabetes care plan for schools (called a 504 plan) at www.diabetes.org.
* **Tell all of your friends.** Whenever someone comes over to your house or every time your parents pick you up at school, have them tell your friends a few things. They should know that if you were ever to "fall asleep" or lose consciousness, they should squirt a little frosting on your gums and get an adult.

They should also know why they must never eat your special food.

* **Have special food at the school.** I always had granola bars and caramels in my desk just in case. I also had my little Igloo cooler under my teacher's desk filled with all sorts of food, so I could recover from a low. I had food like apple juice, snack crackers, more granola bars, caramels, beef jerky, and any other of my favorite foods—no one wants to eat something gross when they have a low blood sugar.
* **Take your cooler on the bus and on all field trips.**
* **Have a granola bar in your pocket during assemblies.**

One of these points that I cannot stress enough is to let all of your friends know that you have diabetes. Tell them what to do when you need sugar.

One day out on the playground, I just sat down and felt really dizzy. My good friend Kevin knew there was something wrong with me. He started talking to me and walked me to the office, called my mom, and started to feed me my caramels. Sometimes no grown-ups are around, and you might feel too bad to go all the way to your cooler or desk, but your friends can always help you.

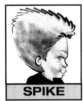

Friends: They're not just for loaning you money anymore.

We gave every teacher and the principal a copy of my symptoms (pages 140–141) and a clear plastic baggie filled with a small Cake Mate frosting, a 6-oz can of apple juice, a granola bar, and peanuts. It helped the teachers know what to do if we got low in class.

## WHAT THE DOC SAYS:

The take-home lesson here is clear: Don't isolate yourself. I've known kids with diabetes who felt embarrassed, ashamed, or just different from everyone else, and therefore, they didn't want to tell others about their condition. While these feelings are understandable, isolating yourself or trying to hide your diabetes is really not in your best interest. First of all, virtually everyone has something that he or she feels this way about, whether it's a physical trait, a personality feature, or just a weird family member. Be proud of who you are and what makes you unique, even your diabetes. When you tell others, you give them a chance to know you better, let them be available if you truly need help (such as if you get low), and may even have a profound effect on them that you could never foresee.

For example, my best friend in junior high school had diabetes, and I truly believe that knowing him and seeing what he had to do to care for himself on a daily basis gave me a deep respect for him and his family. He was one important reason that I eventually became a pediatric endocrinologist. Thank you, Steve.

— MW

## SUPPORT GROUPS

Over the years, we have been involved in playgroups, Kids with Diabetes, Inc., the Ojai Kids, and other support groups, including the PADRE Foundation, the ADA, and the JDRF. It's great to meet with other kids who have diabetes and to share stories and experiences and ideas about how to do things. In fact, that is why we wrote this book—to offer support to other kids with diabetes. Our mom offers the same kind of support to the parents, and we all help each other.

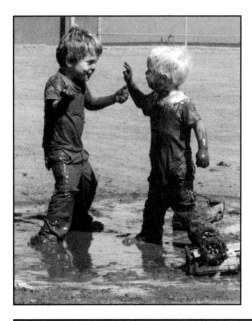

**Spike and Bo, in their natural element.**

## WHAT THE DOC SAYS:

I strongly recommend that you consider finding and joining a diabetes support group for kids or teens. Having a group of people your own age to meet with on a regular basis can provide you with the type of support you need to stay motivated to take care of yourself. We know the benefits of support groups for young people with diabetes, including improved diabetes knowledge, self-care, and communication with parents. Let's face it: we human beings are social animals. We all need some help, guidance, and advice sometimes, and we all need to give some help and guidance, too. You will benefit in more ways than you realize now. To find a group in your area, talk to your health care team, local ADA chapter, or other local diabetes organizations.

# 4 Outdoor School

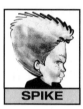

SPIKE

All through elementary school, the one thing Bo and I looked forward to more than anything else was attending Outdoor School. (It's like going to camp with your school. You sleep in a tent or cabin, and you're kind of roughing it.) When it came time to go, though, I thought that I might not be able to make it. I was completely wrong. I was fortunate enough to have my mother come along as a chaperone. If your parents have the time and money, I strongly suggest that they go with you on excursions like these or at least spend a day training a teacher or another parent who will be going. I was extremely grateful that my mother came. Diabetes places a lot of responsibility on all of us kids, and any time that we can be a little freer is extremely valuable.

There were a lot of things to do before heading off to Catalina Island. You can use what we did to plan your own camping or outdoor school experience.

* **Contact the camp beforehand.** Let the supervisors and counselors at any camp you are going to attend know that you have diabetes and give them clear instructions on what to do if you have low blood sugars.

25

* **Look into eating arrangements.** Be sure that there will always be food available and that the people in charge know to give you access whenever necessary.
* **Bring along plenty of extra insulin.** Murphy's Law applies especially well to diabetes. Whenever you mix insulin and backpacks and rocky hikes, chances are something will break. Be sure to bring plenty of extra insulin, syringes, and injection devices or, if you're pumping, infusion sites, reservoirs, batteries, and back-up syringes. Remember to let the camp know before you get there that you will need to refrigerate your insulin. Advance notice always helps.
* **Bring extra food.** Always take your own special snack food; nobody understands what special food you need better than you. Wherever you go, you need extra food, even if it is at a camp

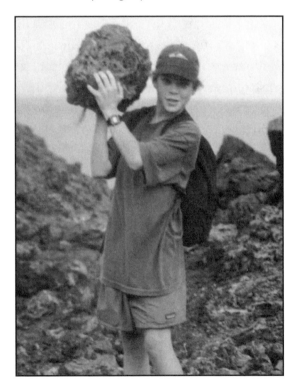

**Spike, acting tough in the Galapagos Islands.**

where they tell you to keep food out of tents because of bears or other scavengers. The counselors will be able to tell you what kind of food and packaging are required to prevent or contain the smells that attract animals. This is another reason for contacting the camp before you go.

* **Be especially careful of cold water.** At Catalina we went for a night snorkel. Despite wearing a full wetsuit—beaver tail and all—I still became excessively cold, and my sugars dropped significantly. It's OK to swim in to shore early. Just tell an adult that you need to go in for food because of your diabetes and be sure to swim in with a friend.

The key thing to do when going to a camp or outdoor school or anything of that nature is to let the people running it know about your special needs well ahead of time. This will help prepare them, and they will help you gain access to anything that you may need while you're there. At Catalina I had to get food out of the cafeteria during "closed time" on several occasions. Everything was fine, though, because everybody knew that I had permission.

For five days of camping on Catalina, I took a small suitcase filled with 1 box each of Wheat Thins, Cheez-Its, and chocolate chip cookies, 3 bottles of Gatorade, 12 granola bars, 5 bags of beef jerky, 1 tub of frosting, 3 tubes of frosting (for my wetsuit), 1 small jar of peanut butter, a jar of peanuts, plastic baggies, paper bags, and a marking pen. Each morning we prepared snacks for 10 a.m., 2 p.m., 4 p.m., and 8 p.m. Then we put them in bags, wrote the snack time on the bag, put them into my backpack, and I was off.

## BO GOES TO CAMP

My friends Rory and Will and I drove up to Big Bear Lake for a work weekend at Camp Conrad-Chinnock. It was a great weekend, even though we forgot to bring sleeping bags and nearly froze. A hundred volunteers arrived with their pickup trucks, toolboxes, and know-how to get the camp ready for the summer. Parents and kids raked leaves, cleaned the pool, and got the craft shack organized. Crews cut down dead pine trees, patched the roof, and built new cabins. Rory, Will, and I hauled rocks and built a dozen bunk beds, and we got to know some sterling people.

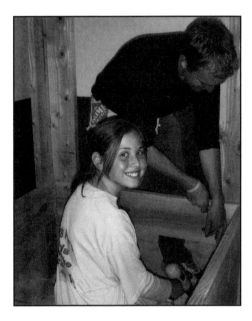

**Abby Stewart and Bo at camp.**

While we were putting the bunks together, Abby Stewart, age twelve, told me how she discovered camp. Here is her story, along with those of some other people from camp.

### Abby's Story

When I was seven years old I went to camp with my whole family. That's where I met my best friend. We were in the same cabin. We had so much fun, and we would never have known each other if it wasn't for camp.

Now I look forward to camp every year. It's on my calendar in big bold letters: Camp Conrad-Chinnock! Camp is not something you want to miss.

Some kids worry that if they go to camp they might miss their parents. Well, you can go to family camp, and your parents and your brothers and sisters will be there too! That's how I started camping—at family camp.

The first time I went to summer camp on my own I was so busy having fun I didn't miss my family one bit. At camp everyone knows about diabetes, so you don't have to explain stuff. You get to talk about everything, like how to deal with stuff at school, and you'll get some ideas from the other kids in your cabin. For example, if you have a question about how you test your blood sugar in class, you have a whole cabin full of kids who have ideas.

I've been going to camp for five years and I really love it. I love making friends, talking about things, swimming, hiking, and making crafts. And the food is really good, too. It's better than home! When I'm old enough I plan to be a counselor, and then I want to work here, because it's a great place. At camp you spend a week with the best people. I'm glad I found out about camp!

## Tracy Fulkerson's Story

I started camping when I was eight years old. I just love it here. I remember how it felt every year when we signed me up for camp—my eyes would light up, and I would look forward to camp all year long. When I was sixteen I became a CIT (counselor in training). I'm twenty-two now and a counselor, and I wouldn't think of missing a summer at camp. Camp serves some magical purpose!

**Matt, the Camp Cook**

I love my summer job working in the kitchen at camp. I do it for the kids, for the looks on their faces...so they can have this wonderful experience!

**Dr. Rocky Wilson**

Kids, search out as many friends as you can who have diabetes... and what better place to meet them than at camp! Camp is a great place to help you figure everything out and build your team. There are lots of ways to get to camp—family camp, work camp, and camp for kids. You can find out about camp at www.dys.org or at www.diabetes.org. Diabetes camp is worldwide!

## WHAT THE DOC SAYS:

I highly recommend an experience in the outdoors, whether at an organized diabetes summer camp or through some other program. For a number of years, I had the privilege of leading teenagers with diabetes into the wilderness on backpacking and whitewater canoeing adventures. Not only can you do these things safely with diabetes, but you may find that "getting away from it all" is a good opportunity to learn how flexible you really can be with your diabetes. The challenges of a different environment offer a great way to learn more about yourself and your diabetes self-care. The best advice about such experiences is to plan ahead. By considering all of your needs and discussing them ahead of time with the camp or program staff, you can set up a situation where you can have a terrific experience in the great outdoors.

# 5 Sports

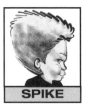

**SPIKE**

When I first found out that I had something called diabetes, I was afraid that my short-lived sports career had, perhaps, come to an early end. This couldn't have been any further from the truth. With only very minor alterations to my schedule, I was able to continue playing soccer, baseball, and basketball, so diabetes didn't affect my abilities one bit. Bo and I were still able to make the all-star teams for soccer and baseball (I was never any good at basketball to begin with).

## TEAM SPORTS

Here are some of the things that kids with diabetes have to do a little differently when playing team sports:

* **Just like at school, tell everyone involved: coaches, players, other parents, even referees.** Diabetes is certainly nothing to be ashamed of—it can't keep you from doing anything—and definitely not something to keep a secret.
* **Check your blood sugar before each practice and each game.** If you have low blood sugar, do not start playing. Exercise lowers your sugar fairly rapidly, so you need to eat and start feel-

ing better before you start to play. (It should only take 5 or 10 minutes to get your sugar up.) You also shouldn't go out on the field if your sugar is very high (above 300 mg/dl). It seems logical to get exercise to help bring your sugars down, but very high blood sugars and exercise just make you feel bad. Take a little insulin, one or two units (very little—it's better to be high than low), and eat a little. **Always eat something when you take insulin, even when you are high.** Test again in 15 minutes to see if you've lowered your blood sugar enough to play.

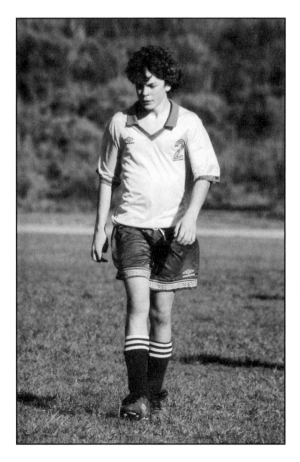

**Spike, tired after a soccer match.**

* **During breaks in the game, quarters, innings, and half time, eat a little something.** I always drink Gatorade at quarters and maybe eat a little granola bar at halftime. You don't have to come out of a game to eat; just run to the sideline. Tell the referee what you are doing and there won't be any problems.
* **Sometimes you need to eat some real food.** If you are playing just after a big meal and just took insulin or if you are getting lots of exercise, you may need to eat a meal between or even during your game. I always liked McDonald's Chicken Mc-Nuggets because you can eat them one at a time. Your friends might beg you for some (especially if it's been a long tournament), but just tell them that you have to eat it, and they will understand.

The three best ways of controlling diabetes are with insulin, diet, and exercise. Your blood sugar may be a little bit wacky when you start playing a sport after a month or more off, but soon your athletic activities will help bring your sugars down to a totally normal level. By just being a little bit more careful and by eating a little bit more than you used to, you can play as many sports as you like and may be an all-star in every one of them!

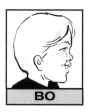 Especially if you're taller than your older brother!

## WHAT THE DOC SAYS:

Spike and Bo are right on. Diabetes will not keep you from participating in sports or other activities. To get the most from your sports activities, you'll need to check your blood sugar before and after you exercise to see the effect of exercise on your blood sugar. If you have 1/2–1 hour before an athletic event, you could eat a granola bar for the carbohydrates. If it is two hours before the game, you could have a low-fat, moderate-protein, high-carbohydrate meal, such as cereal, banana, and milk for breakfast or pizza and salad for lunch or dinner. A turkey or chicken sandwich would work well, too. The carbohydrates in these meals will be working just about the time you are playing.

If you are going to play strenuously for an hour or less, a box of juice (8 oz) or Gatorade should keep your blood sugar up. A good rule of thumb is that carbohydrates raise your blood sugar for the first 1–2 hours, protein for the next 2–4 hours, and fat for the 4–6 hours after the food is eaten. McDonald's McNuggets, like most fast foods, are very high in fat, so try to eat an amount that fits into your meal plan.

Remember that exercise makes your body more sensitive to insulin, so you may get low blood sugars immediately after exercise and also later on, when your insulin action is peaking. So, it is wise to take an extra bedtime snack or snack bar with cornstarch on the days that you get lots of exercise.

Check your blood sugar before the game. If it is 100 mg/dl or less, have 15 g of carbohydrate right away and again every hour. If it is 170 mg/dl, have 15 g of carbohydrate in an hour and again every hour. If it is 200 mg/dl, go ahead and play, but check your blood sugar every hour. If it is 240 mg/dl, check your urine for ketones and, if there are none present, then go ahead and play, checking your blood sugar every hour.

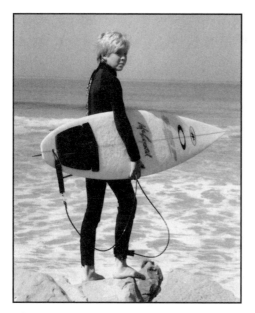

Bo ready to surf at Pitas Point.

## SURFING

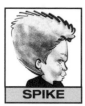

SPIKE

Bo and I have surfed since we were six years old. It is my favorite sport and also the one where I have run into the most hurdles due to diabetes. The generally cold waters of Ventura County are especially draining on my body, and I have found that even with a wetsuit, it is not wise to stay out in the line-up for much more than an hour before having a little snack. Your body burns a lot of calories when you're paddling your heart out (feels like for your life—sometimes it is) in ocean water that's barely 50 degrees.

Here are some things I do now to avoid the lows:

\* **Stock up on fast food every single time I go to the beach.** Always eat a burger or a taco before paddling out and each time you paddle back in. It takes a lot of energy for anyone to surf all day.

* **Roll up a tube of frosting in the sleeve of your wetsuit.** If you ever have a severe low while in the water, a tube of frosting can be what it takes to get you back in to shore.

* **Take a cooler.** Filling a cooler full of food and bringing it to the beach can save you a lot of money at McDonald's and Taco Bell. I still recommend buying and eating some protein-filled food before you paddle out, though. Keep a glucagon kit in your cooler.

* **Never stay out in the line-up for more than an hour.** Even if it's the best surf you have ever seen, you need to go in and eat frequently. This will ensure that you are feeling great and can surf your best on the best days. If you're pumping you'll need to paddle in just as often to check your sugar and to plug in for a little bit of insulin. You don't want to go a long time with no insulin in your system at all, so paddling in every hour for just a fraction of a unit is a good idea.

* **If you feel low, tell someone you are surfing with.** If you have diabetes, never surf alone. There is too much potential for getting into trouble. If you ever feel low when you're out in the water, just tell your friend or even a complete stranger if he or she is the only one around who can help you get in.

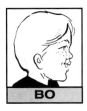

I have never actually passed out in the surf, but I have had some scary moments. After a rather large wipe-out and at least ten seconds under the surface, I paddled back out past the breakers. I was pretty cold and figured that was why I was shaking so much. Then my leg began to cramp up something fierce, but I rubbed it, and about three minutes later, I had control of it again. I was shaking pretty good by now and could hardly hold my head off the board. I had enough sense to turn toward shore and start paddling, so the white-water washed me in. I left my board on the beach, climbed the stairs to my friend's beach house, and started eating ice cream. I didn't feel normal for more than an hour and a full meal or two later. I thought I was just cold, but my mom told me that after I had come in, she had tested my blood sugar, and it was a scant 20 mg/dl. I was pretty lucky, but I wish that I had had enough sense to just tell somebody out in the line-up.

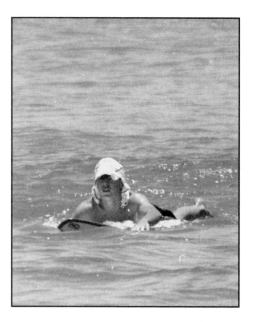

**Spike, paddling in, Baja, Mexico.**

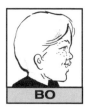

I learned a lesson that day: if you are feeling funny or bad, tell somebody.

Life offers you many exciting, fun, and adventuresome experiences. You can do them all with diabetes, but please take the time to think ahead, and don't dismiss the risks of certain activities just because you don't want to be different. The advice in this section shows a nice balance between adventure and reasonable precautions, and you can apply it to other adventurous activities. Plan ahead, and don't be afraid or embarrassed to ask for help if you need it. Sometimes we think we have to do things on our own or else somehow we've failed. In fact, we all depend on each other in some way or other, so if you get into a difficult situation in the surf, or on a mountain, or wherever you find yourself, just ask for help.

## MOTORCYCLE AND BICYCLE RIDING

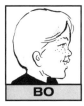

BO

Motorcycle riding is a unique sport. There is more than just physical exertion involved. It takes a lot of mental and physical work to ride for long periods of time. It can be really cold or really hot out, and because you can travel so far on a bike, you must be prepared.

Spike and I follow this routine for both motorcycle and bicycle riding.

✳ **Pack food.** The most important thing to remember is to take enough food when you go for a ride. For instance, if you are going out for a two-hour ride, one hour down the trail and one hour back, you have to be prepared to be able to walk back. It may be miles. Plan for the worst. Take enough food with you in your butt pack so that if your bike breaks down or if you have a wreck, you can get back to civilization. Take a glucagon kit. I always carry a large butt pack.

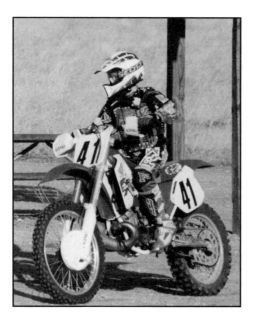

**Bo, riding in
the desert.**

* **Check your sugar before you start riding.** You may also want to reduce your insulin when you're riding.

* **Calorie up before riding.** I find that I can eat twice as much as usual when I'm riding all day, because the sport uses so much energy.

* **Try a Camelbak.** For any long rides, you'll appreciate a Camelbak to carry liquids. It's a small backpack that holds liquids with a long straw to your mouth so you can drink while you're riding.

* **Never ride alone.** If your bike won't make it back, you can always hop on your buddy's bike and get a ride back. My friends always carry a tube of frosting with them just in case I get low, and I'm not in shape to help myself. The frosting perks you up enough to eat a real snack.

* **Prepare for accidents and injury.** If you should have an accident that requires a ride to the hospital, you'll have your kit and snack food right with you in your butt pack.

* **Know what to do at the hospital.** If you should have to go to the hospital, take your kit filled with your insulin and your meter kit with your blood testing stuff. Pumpers, take your pump supplies, extra infusion sites, and reservoirs. Things will go much more smoothly if you and your parents monitor your blood sugar while the doctor takes care of stitches or broken bones. Injuries can cause your sugar to soar or crash—usually crash.

## BO'S MOTORCYCLE ACCIDENT

It was January 17, 1994, the day of the big Northridge quake, here in Southern California. After the excitement of the earthquake, I went for a trail ride. I was taking it easy on my bike, just going up a hill in some soft dirt when I simply laid the bike over. The chain caught my leg, cutting through my jeans from knee to ankle. It splayed my shin open, a six-inch gash to the bone. I was able to ride home to get help.

On the way to the hospital, I had my butt pack with my kit and snacks. We tested my blood sugar in the car. It dropped a little,

> **WHAT THE DOC SAYS:**
>
> Long bicycle rides do use up a lot of calories. You should stop, on average, every hour to eat something and continue on. Make certain you carry plenty of carbohydrate-containing snacks. If you feel low, don't wait for a scenic view to stop and eat. Stop immediately and eat a fast-acting sugar food, and then eat something that lasts longer. Check your blood sugar before beginning and whenever you stop to be sure you are eating enough snacks. Insulin pumps are helpful for long-distance exercise. In these instances, you will not take a bolus and can adjust your basal rates.

and I needed some of that snack. In the emergency room, while the doctor irrigated my wound and got ready to sew it up, my mom used my kit to keep testing my blood to monitor my blood sugar. She gave me food and Gatorade when I needed it. We probably did three blood tests during the emergency room visit. My sugar kept dropping, and I kept eating and drinking.

## BACKPACKING

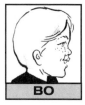
BO

Backpacking is a lot of fun, but there are a few extra things you need to take with you and a few things you need to know. You need to take extra food, so you have enough to make it if you get lost or end up spending more time away from civilization than you planned. Spike and I always carry food for an additional 24 hours. Remember, when you are out in the woods away from people, stores, and medical care, you will need to take extra precautions. Do not hike alone. Tell someone where you will be, protect your kit so that nothing gets broken banging around in your backpack, and carry extra insulin. Don't exhaust yourself, do eat frequently, and filter the water. You don't need to get sick.

Besides warm clothes and water, here's what I pack:

* **Granola bars.** Put them in your backpack and in your pockets, where they are easy to reach.
* **Gatorade.** This is a good drink for low blood sugars. It is also a good way to keep your body hydrated while hiking or backpacking. You can carry Gatorade in a powder form; then all you have to do is add water. It's lighter to carry the powder.
* **Beef jerky and peanuts.** Jerky is lightweight and a good source of protein. Jerky and peanuts are good long-acting foods to have when you'll be using up lots of energy.

* **Trail mix.** Make sure you don't abuse trail mix. Trail mix often has a lot of chocolate, raisins, and other dried fruit mixed in. These can be good for low blood sugars but shouldn't be eaten freely. Be aware of what is in your trail mix, and stay away from the ones that are packed with sweets.
* **Kit.** Keep your kit out of the sun. Keep it cool if the weather is hot, or warm if you're hiking in the snow. If you're camping in the snow, sleep with it in your sleeping bag.
* **Glucagon.** Carry your glucagon kit. Tell your friends to inject you with glucagon if you should pass out and the frosting doesn't work. Make sure they know exactly where it is or let them carry it. There is no 911 out in the wilderness.

Although I highly recommend getting plenty of exercise, backpacking requires some preparation. You use extreme amounts of energy, especially when you're at high altitudes, when you're carrying a heavy pack, or when it's cold. Before you go backpacking, think about these things:

* **Calories.** You may need up to twice as many calories when backpacking.
* **Never hike alone.** Hike with a friend. Friends can help carry the extra food you'll need.
* **Reduce your insulin.** Start out using less insulin. If it's a serious trip, you will use less insulin. I usually inject or bolus only half of my regular short-acting dose before a day of backpacking. Check your blood sugar often. This way you'll know what you need to eat and how much insulin you should inject.
* **Snacks.** Pack snacks in separate bags and write the time to eat the snack on each bag. When you change your routine, sometimes you forget to eat. This will help you remember.

## WHAT THE DOC SAYS:

Backpacking into the wilderness can be a life-changing experience that will challenge you to be your best and give you many rewards. But it does add many variables to your usual diabetes self-care plan with which you may not be familiar. I would offer the following practical tips based on my personal experiences in the backcountry with teens with diabetes.

1. With the increased activity, temperature extremes, and high altitude often found in the backcountry, hypoglycemia is quite common. Be prepared to check your sugar frequently, including late at night or maybe even in the middle of the night, especially if you've spent a long day hiking. Carry plenty of "low food" to treat hypoglycemia. This could be raisins, dried fruit, nutrition bars, or glucose tablets. Keep your gear well organized, and always know where the low foods are.

2. Be very knowledgeable about your diabetes, or go with someone who is knowledgeable. Such variables as extreme exercise, altitude, or climate mean you may need to significantly change your usual insulin dose rapidly. Having to reduce your insulin dose by 20–50% is not unusual.

3. If you go to high altitudes too quickly, you may experience symptoms of altitude sickness, which can mimic low blood sugar. Drink plenty of water to prevent dehydration. Drink even before you are thirsty.

4. Since you may be far from conventional medical care, know basic first aid, or travel with someone who does.

5. Some glucose meters don't work as well at high altitudes. Check with the manufacturer before you leave home.

6. Never, ever, hike alone. A low blood sugar on the trail should not turn a wonderful experience in nature into a disaster.

7. Always carry some form of identification stating that you have diabetes and an instructional sheet on what to do if you can't help yourself.

Warm muscles use up sugar independent of insulin. After a day of heavy exercise, your muscles will continue to use sugar for hours. You will need to use far less short-acting insulin at dinner. Be prepared to wake up and check a midnight blood sugar level, and watch for lower blood sugar levels for the 24 hours after you return home.

## MORE ABOUT HEAVY EXERCISE

We are talking about hard, prolonged exercise. Heavy exercise is a day of sports tournaments, snowboarding or skiing all day, racquetball, surfing for three hours or more, motorcycle riding all day, or bike riding half a day. It also applies to an afternoon of high school practice for active sports like football, basketball, swim team, soccer, or track. (This doesn't apply to a game of pick-up basketball in the driveway.) Here are some important tips:

* **Lower your dinnertime insulin dose after you've done extreme exercise.** You will also want to adjust your insulin dose down before heavy exercise. When you have diabetes and you exercise all day, you will need to stop and think about just how much short-acting insulin you should take at dinner. Each sport you play will have slightly different calorie and insulin requirements.
* **Exhaustion calls for a different routine.** This is because all day your muscles have been using up the sugar from your meals. The sugar that was stored in your muscle tissue has been used up, too. For the next eight hours or so, in the middle of the night, while you are sleeping, your muscles will be taking sugar out of your blood stream and putting it back into storage. Low blood sugar can result.

After exercising all day, you need to avoid getting drastically low in the middle of the night. Eat dinner, cut down your insulin dose by 1/2 or more, and eat a good snack with protein and carbs before going to sleep. (Eat a snack before bed even if your sugar is a little high, because your warm muscles will use it up during the night.)

Think about a soccer game. Soccer is a running game. You might run three or four miles during a soccer game. If it's a morning game and I usually take eight units of short-acting insulin, I'll take only four units. After the game, at lunchtime I'll test. If I usually take five units of short-acting insulin at lunch, I'll only take two. By dinnertime, after a morning game, I'll test and take my normal dose.

Now consider a soccer tournament. You might have three soccer games on the same day with more games to come on the next day. You might run eight or ten miles on a tournament day. Before the first game, I cut my insulin dose in half. I snack at quarters, and at halftime. I have a huge lunch and test. If my sugar is low, I skip my noontime insulin. I continue snacking and eating for energy throughout game two and game three.

## WHAT THE DOC SAYS:

Exercise lowers blood sugar independently of insulin. This effect can be so great with extreme exercise that some diabetic professional athletes will take only extremely small insulin doses before a big game. The actual effect of heavy exercise on blood sugar can differ greatly from person to person, and the increase in glucose use following exercise can last for several days. Whatever changes you make in your insulin dose to compensate for exercise, be sure to test your sugar afterward to learn about how your body responds when you push it. If you have any questions, be sure to ask your diabetes health care professional.

By dinnertime my sugar might be climbing. Let's say it's around 180 mg/dl. But after heavy exercise your dinnertime insulin dose will be different. It will be lower. I will cut down my short-acting insulin dose to half or less.

# 6 Pursuing Academics

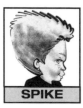

**SPIKE**

Diabetes doesn't have to affect your academic schoolwork as long as you keep even moderate control of it. I was able to become the valedictorian of my high school and get a 1550 on my SAT. (I would like to point out for the record that I got this score when the maximum was 1600 points, not 2400 points like it is today—thank you very much.) Diabetes in no way challenged my academics. A few precautions can be taken, however, to ensure that it doesn't hamper you in your schooling.

Some things to do to keep your scores up:

* **Always bring extra food and snacks when taking major tests** (finals, SAT, AP). I typically bring a granola bar or two and a bottle of Gatorade to snack on while testing and a whole snack (crackers, string cheese, banana) to eat during the breaks in the tests.
* **Inform the test proctor of your needs.** Some of the tests have specific instructions against eating. If you tell the administrator that you have diabetes and don't make a big deal out of eating, there won't be a problem. If there is a problem, you don't have to take the test, and you can notify the test administrators. You do have to be treated a little differently sometimes.

* **Remember to eat.** Even if you don't feel low, you should "graze." You may think it strange, but strenuous brain activity actually has the same effect on my sugar as physical activities. My sugars drop significantly when I compete or test without eating. Don't worry if other students are not allowed to eat in test situations; you basically have to.

* **If you feel low during a test, inform your teacher or the test administrator.** In the classroom, your teacher will already know you have diabetes, so you will probably be able to retake the test. At standardized national tests, you may have to contact the testing center for information regarding their policy, but you are entitled to a retake.

* **Let your teacher know.** If you were having low sugars or working on getting rid of ketones and it kept you from doing your homework, let your teacher know the next day. Never use diabetes as an excuse if it didn't really affect anything, but if it did, don't be afraid to tell your teacher. They know that your health is more important than one assignment and will undoubtedly let you make it up.

If you feel bad, always remember to take care of your health before anything else, even final exams. If you can't make up a test, remember that a grade is just a mark on a piece of paper. Five years down the road it won't mean a thing, but the way you feel will. I can count on one hand the times that I have had to stop doing something academic because of my blood sugar. Diabetes may give you tiny setbacks, but it can't keep you from any kind of scholarly achievement whatsoever.

## WHAT THE DOC SAYS:

This section raises interesting issues regarding diabetes and special treatment. While diabetes may not be a disability in the classic use of the word, the reality is that there may be certain circumstances where special treatment is a medical necessity. My best advice is to be realistic about your situation and ask only for what you truly need. Don't use your diabetes to manipulate situations falsely in your favor. The balanced approach suggested in this section will serve you well.

# 7 Eating Out

Going out to dinner really isn't much different at all when you have diabetes. As in most other activities, though, you'll need to be a little more responsible. You can still eat most everything on the menu—just stay away from too much food with lots of sugar and match your carbohydrates with protein (see pages 135–137). When you go out to dinner, you might as well treat yourself to something you enjoy.

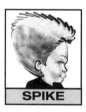
SPIKE

Here are some tips I follow when I go out to dinner:

✻ **Never shoot up or bolus too early.** You want to make sure food will be available when you need it. At restaurants, you never know how long it will take before you are served. To avoid lows, I take my insulin after the food arrives. Ideally, you should shoot up about 5–30 minutes before you eat (depending on what type of insulin you take), but at restaurants that's impossible to gauge. Sometimes, if I have high blood sugar, I inject my insulin a few minutes after ordering my food but even that is taking a chance. What if they lose my order?

* **Don't be afraid to tell your waiter that you absolutely must have some food.** If you shot up too early or are just having a low for other reasons, tell the waiter that you have diabetes and need food right away. Maybe you can tip a little extra (don't worry about that until after your sugar has come back up).

* **Always bring a little bit of your own food.** When you are going out to eat, you should still carry your trusty granola bar in your pocket. This will keep you from having to demand food and will allow you to shoot up earlier. If your food is long in coming, you will have some backup right there.

* **Watch your sugar.** Restaurants load any sweet food with tons of extra sugar. Desserts are a luxury, not a necessity, so I avoid them most of the time and maybe have a bite of my date's or my friend's. On very special occasions, I sometimes treat myself, but I don't usually eat a whole dessert. After avoiding sugar for so long, I noticed that really sweet things lose their appeal—kind of a plus when you have diabetes or just want to be healthy.

* **Don't be shy about shooting up or testing.** I have known some people with diabetes who hide their injections out of some notion of politeness. Don't be afraid to shoot up at the table. You can do it without attracting a lot of attention. I sometimes set up my meter right on my lap if I'm feeling bashful and test without anyone noticing. Or you may want to ask if anyone is squeamish and tell them what you are doing. Most people are extremely interested and even mesmerized by it. I try to get my friends to do it for me. I draw the insulin; then they can inject in my arms and give my legs and hips a break. Testing goes the same way.

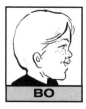

BO

Just remember to go ahead and tell people that you have diabetes. Shoot up only when you know food is coming, and then eating out will be a cinch!

## WHAT THE DOC SAYS:

The best lesson here is, again, don't be shy about who you are and what you need to do to care for yourself. Next, even if you are very knowledgeable about nutrition and are great at counting carbs (see pages 128–129), it can be pretty tricky to estimate the carbohydrate content or portion sizes of restaurant food. Do your best, but be prepared to supplement with extra insulin if you undershoot the insulin dose.

# 8 Traveling with Your Family

The time to be most careful is when you are far away from home and far away from people who know you have diabetes and know what to do. You must be more careful, but you can still have the time of your life traveling around the country and the world. As long as you take a few precautions and pack a little bit extra, you can avoid any real problems.

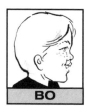

BO

Plan ahead to be safe when traveling. Here's what Spike and I do:

* **Pack lots of extra insulin and other diabetes supplies.** I usually pack my normal kit (page 11) and then pack one or two more duplicate kits (depending on the duration of my trip and how far I'm going). You shouldn't put all of your extra insulin in the same place though, because if one bottle is lost, stolen, or broken, then all of them will be too.

* **Always carry your insulin on you when you fly.** The luggage compartments on many flights either get extremely cold or hot or both, and this is not a good thing for insulin, especially when you are going to be out of the country for a week or two.

* **Let the management at all hotels know that you need to use a freezer for your ice packs.** I always freeze extra ice packs and keep one with my insulin. I don't put my insulin in refrigerators in a hotel kitchen because of the chance that it may be lost, broken, or stolen. You can always buy more ice packs though. Also, try to get a room with a mini bar refrigerator. They work perfectly for insulin.

* **Let the flight attendant on any flight know that you have diabetes.** This way you will be assured of food when you need it, and it is always nice to have some extra peanuts. You can request a special meal several days before you fly, but ask what it will be in case you don't like the food choices.

* **Pharmacies have to give you insulin and needles.** If a pharmacy has what you need in stock, you don't need a prescription to get it. If you are totally without your insulin, syringes, or blood sugar testing equipment, tell the pharmacist that it is an emergency, and he or she will help you out. Show identification that you have diabetes and, if necessary, be stubborn until you get what you need. It's a good idea to have a letter from your doctor or a prescription form stating that you have diabetes and what you need. Be aware that insulin in other countries is not the same potency as ours. You'll have to adjust and inject a different amount to the get the effect you need if you use the syringes that you bring with you. Syringes are different sizes in other countries, too. Ask your doctor for help with this.

* **Take lots of food with you wherever you go.** When I go on big trips, I take an extra suitcase just for food. I take enough beef jerky, Gatorade, crackers, and granola bars to live off for the entire trip if need be. It's a bit of a hassle, but I think I would probably do it now even if I didn't have diabetes. (I like to eat.)

**✳ Carry a glucagon kit.** Also carry directions for how to use it.
**✳ Wear a medical ID and carry a diabetes ID card.**

It is especially important to always have food on you. On our flight home from South Africa, the flight attendants' union was on strike. The in-flight meal consisted of a bag of peanuts and water for a 15-hour flight. That could have been a very bad thing, but Bo and I had plenty of food in our backpacks, so there was no problem at all. On another trip, our truck broke down in the jungles of Costa Rica. We were stuck out in the middle of nowhere for 24 hours. Once again we had well-stocked backpacks, which saved the day. You can avoid serious problems. If you just plan things out wisely and are always prepared for the worst, you can go anywhere and have as much fun as anyone else.

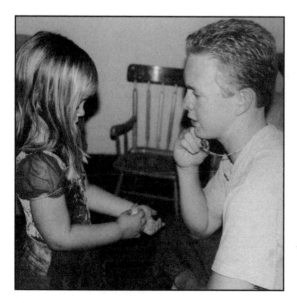

**Bo and Laura, comparing their medical IDs.**

In addition to carrying extra food and diabetes supplies with you at all times while traveling, you have to adjust to time changes. Move meals back or forward a few hours at a time. If there is a large time difference, take extra short-acting insulin to cover highs and take your intermediate-acting insulin at the times you would normally take it—before breakfast, before dinner, or whenever, but use the time of your final destination. For example, if you are traveling from Chicago to London, you would take your pre-dinner insulin in Chicago, take short-acting insulin while flying, and take a pre-breakfast intermediate-acting insulin on London time. For an insulin pump, you just have to give your boluses before eating.

## THE BACKPACK

This is what we carry in our backpacks when we travel. Always keep your insulin and food with you in your backpack.

The main body of the backpack contains:
* insulin kit (page 11)
* meter kit (page 12)
* pumpers: carry extra pump supplies, infusion sets, reservoirs, and inserter
* Gatorade
* 1 box crackers
* 1 box cookies
* jerky
* snacks packed in brown paper bags
* jacket
* hat
* book

The side pocket contains:

* glucagon kit
* frosting
* Imodium—for diarrhea
* Compazine, Phenergan, or
  Tigan—for nausea
  (Compazine is not for children)

* Ketostix
* Tylenol
* Neosporin

The inside pocket contains:

* passport
* tickets

* money

The large front pocket contains:

* toothbrush
* Chapstick
* deodorant
* razor
* swimmer's ear drops or
  ear plugs

* sunscreen lotion
* special medical supplies,
  for example, asthma
  medication
* pens
* small notebook

## WHAT THE DOC SAYS:

Always carry some form of identification stating that you
have diabetes and an instruction sheet on what to do if
you can't help yourself—for example, how to use the
cake frosting or the glucagon.

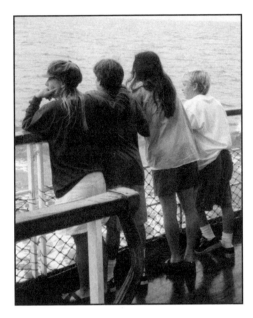

**Jenny, Spike, Mary, and Bo, cruising in the Galapagos.**

## THE FULL MEDICAL KIT

When we go on a big trip, say, surfing to Costa Rica, we carry a full medical kit. Ours contains:

* first aid cream and first aid guide
* Benadryl—for allergies
* antiseptic spray
* Ibuprofen—for pain and inflammation
* Dramamine—for motion sickness
* Band-Aids
* rolled tourniquet
* tweezers
* antiseptic cream—for cuts
* cold sore cream
* instant ice pack
* swimmer's ear drops—preventative
* bee sting kit

* gauze pads
* scissors
* needle and thread

We also carry the following prescription drugs:

* glucagon kit
* hydrocortisone cream—anti-inflammatory, for rashes
* antipyrine/benzocaine otic—for ear pain
* Cortisporin Otic—for pain, infection, inflammation
* Lomotil—anti-diarrhea, can be taken up to four times a day
  (Imodium is available over the counter.)
* Compazine or Phenergan—anti-nausea
* Keflex—for upper respiratory infection, skin abrasions
* Tobrex—for eye infection
* Vicodin—for stingray or jellyfish stings

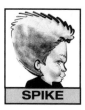

**SPIKE**

Immerse stingray wounds in hot water, as hot as you can stand, to neutralize the toxin. Ammonia can also neutralize the acid in the toxin, so you might carry a small bottle. When you are out in the boonies, put urine on a jellyfish sting.

## WHAT THE DOC SAYS:

You can carry different brands of medical supplies in your backpack; just be sure that they do what you expect them to do. For example, Neosporin Plus is an antibiotic cream to keep cuts from getting infected. Talk with your doctor about which drugs—both over-the-counter and prescription—you might want to carry with you.

# 9 Driving

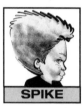

Driving gives everyone tremendous freedom, especially people with diabetes. No longer must you carry a cooler—you can keep one in your car. No longer must you worry constantly about getting an ice pack—you can have a mobile refrigeration unit. No longer must you worry about where your next meal will come from—you can drive down the block to a fast-food place or store. As long as you are a bit more responsible and never get behind the wheel when you are low, being able to drive can help make your diabetes an even smaller inconvenience.

I have never personally experienced any real lows or scary incidents while driving, and neither has Bo. However, I realize that the potential for accidents as a result of an insulin reaction is real, and so I take all the necessary precautions. I'd like to think that it is my wariness that has kept things running smoothly.

Driving comes with added freedoms and added responsibilities. Here are some tips to keep in mind:

* **Never drive with low blood sugar.** If you drive while very low, you might as well be driving drunk. You will be sluggish, slow to react, and simply asking for trouble. Instead, either get a friend to drive you to a food source or eat some of the food

you have in your vehicle and wait until it takes effect before you drive anywhere.

* **Keep a refrigeration device (or cooler) in your vehicle.** I have an electric cooler that plugs into my cigarette lighter. There is plenty of room for my kit, extra insulin, and food such as Gatorade, granola bars, peanuts, jerky, and anything else I may feel like eating. This is the single greatest benefit of always having my truck around—independence from always carrying lots of food on my person and always trying to find a refrigerator.

* **Don't worry about leaving a social event momentarily to get food.** If mealtime rolls around and you need to eat, now you can go get food whenever you like. Having your own vehicle makes your life a little more private. You no longer have to plan out your whole day or make a fuss over needing to eat. I still recommend telling people where you are going, in case you're lower than you think and you end up needing someone to come looking for you.

* **Don't be afraid to pull off the road if you are not feeling right.** Pull over, have a drink of Gatorade, test your sugar, and either shoot up or eat if you need to. This is what emergency-only stopping places are for.

* **Be extra prepared on long drives.** When I drive home from college, I'm on the road for at least five or six hours. I always keep a bottle of Gatorade, several granola bars, and a big bag of chips on the seat next to me in case I start feeling low between fast-food stops. I also keep jerky there, so I can have a low-carb snack if I get hungry.

* **Carry a card in your wallet that identifies you as having diabetes.** Keep it right next to your license. This way if you get pulled over for suspected drunken driving (which may happen if you don't realize that you are low), the officer will realize that

you need sugar and possibly further medical attention. Also, if you are in an accident, the paramedics will know that you need special attention.

* **Wear a medical ID bracelet or necklace.**

## WHAT THE DOC SAYS:

Never get into a car, either as a driver or as a passenger, when you feel low. Always eat or drink a rapid-acting sugar food first and then eat a longer-acting snack. Check your sugar before beginning to drive and don't drive until your blood sugar is at least 80–100 mg/dl. If driving alone, make sure that you have a rapid-acting sugar food or drink and a snack on the seat next to you, so you can reach them easily. Most important of all, don't wait to eat when you feel low. Stop the car right away, eat, and don't start driving again until your blood sugar is in the safe range. As you do in treating all lows, drink a juice box or take cake frosting or glucose tablets to raise your blood sugar levels rapidly, and then eat a granola bar or half a sandwich—food with carbohydrates and protein in it.

Remember to wear a medical ID bracelet or necklace when driving. This will increase the likelihood that you will be appropriately treated with glucose if you get low. This also will help you avoid being mistakenly charged with "driving under the influence" (DUI).

# 10 Partying

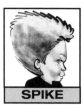

**SPIKE**

When you get into your mid-teens, chances are that you'll be invited to some parties, and chances are that not all of them will be alcohol and drug free. You have to be especially careful with drugs of any kind. And, when you choose not to use them, having diabetes is a perfect excuse to use against peer pressure. Bo and I have found that our friends respect our wishes when we tell them we are not going to drink because of diabetes—I am sure yours will, too.

Here's what to do at a party:

* **Don't drink much at all.** You really shouldn't drink alcohol at all, but if you do, only drink a little. Some alcoholic beverages are full of sugar, so drinking a beer is like drinking a regular Coke. This will cause your sugar to rise and then fall rapidly when it wears off. If you do drink, be sure to eat as well, so you have something to stabilize your sugar. Never drink enough to get drunk and pass out. This is the worst possible scenario. If you pass out and forget to eat or even forget to inject or bolus, you are asking for trouble.

* **Tell your friends to watch out for you.** If you are drinking, make sure someone knows what to do if you pass out, such as give you sugar and call your mom and dad immediately.
* **Don't use tobacco.** Nicotine causes problems with the tiny blood vessels in your arms and legs, and diabetes does that, too. Smoking for even a short period of time damages your circulation, and you want to keep your blood vessels healthy all the time. Who wants to smoke anyway?
* **Be a designated driver.** I drive my friends around and stay completely sober at parties 95% of the time. This is another good way to handle peer pressure. It's always fun to be sober and laugh at all your friends anyway.

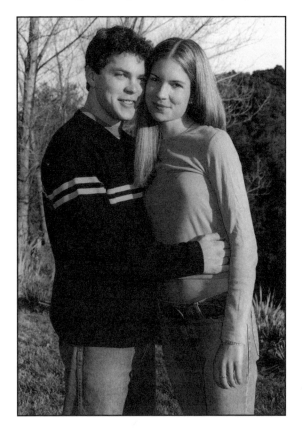

**Spike and Vanessa on a college date.**

* **Whatever you choose to do, do it in moderation.** If you drink, don't drink a six-pack. If you smoke (I don't know why you would want to), only smoke a cigarette or two at parties and nowhere else. Avoid marijuana; it's illegal and can get you into trouble. If you do try marijuana, be careful; only take a couple of hits. The munchies can get you into trouble, but if you pass out and don't eat at all, you will get into worse trouble.

* **Don't be afraid to call your mom and dad and tell them that you aren't feeling well.** This is a good idea for anyone, but it is truly important for people with diabetes.

## WHAT THE DOC SAYS:

Although you may be tired of hearing adults telling you to "Just say no," you need to know that cigarettes, alcohol, and drugs do pose definite serious risks if you have diabetes, over and above the risks they pose for people who don't have diabetes. Spike and Bo give balanced, responsible, and realistic guidelines for you to use in situations where you may find yourself tempted by these substances. Know the facts, and know the risks that you face, particularly on account of your diabetes. The biggest risk from the diabetes perspective is that an altered mental state due to alcohol or drugs can cause you to miss the warning signs of low blood sugar, which may result in a seizure or coma. Also, alcohol can cause low blood sugar, especially if you don't eat while you drink. Cigarettes add to the risk of heart attacks, strokes, and other disorders for which diabetes already increases the risk. Smoking also increases the risk of eye and kidney complications. We all know these substances have the risk of addiction and bad effects on overall health in the long run. Be smart. Use your head and save your heart for better things.

You have to know your limits. Getting addicted to any of these substances will lead to extremely serious consequences for you, and it truly isn't worth it. Just remember that if you choose to try one of these substances, you must eat, too. A high blood sugar is much better than a low one. However, if you choose to avoid these things altogether, diabetes offers you the perfect reason.

# 11 Starting College

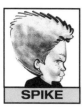
**SPIKE**

I recently graduated from Stanford University. Diabetes didn't affect me any differently in college than it did in high school, but before entering college, I made some special arrangements. Housing plans and meal plans are two parts of college life that need your particular attention.

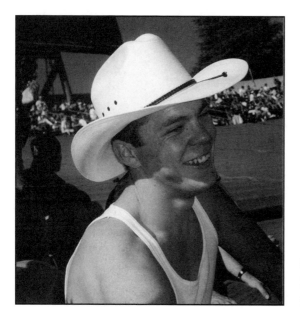

**Spike at a Stanford football game.**

Here's what to do during the enrollment process:

* **Mark the "handicapped" or "chronically ill" box on your applications.** This will let the school know that you have a condition that requires special attention, and this will start the process.
* **Register at the disabilities office.** Diabetes isn't truly a disability, as it can't keep you from doing a single thing, but registering will allow you to get special housing and meal plans. These aren't totally necessary, but they will make your life much easier.
* **Get housing that has a kitchen or is near 24-hour food.** Either get a dorm with a late-night cafeteria or housing that is near fast-food places or eating clubs on campus. You never know when you will have a late-night low. You will need at least a small snack after each late-night study session, so there is no point in making it hard on yourself and having to walk miles to get food.
* **Get a meal plan that has no absolute limit.** The college has to offer you as much food as you need, and you really should get a plan that allows this, even if you have to pay extra.

After you arrive on campus:

* **Keep a drawer stocked with food in your room.** Make sure you tell your friends that it is your special diabetes drawer. You may have to tell them several times before they stop trying to sneak a few cookies and crackers from you while you aren't looking!
* **Put a small refrigerator in your dorm room.** I don't recommend this as a substitute for housing near food but as a complement to it. At school I snacked out of my refrigerator almost nightly to keep my sugars up, and I don't know what I would have done without one.
* **Take any advantages that come your way.** At many schools, if you are registered as having diabetes, they will have someone

take notes for you at any class you miss for medical reasons. They also must allow you to make up any tests missed for that reason. Some schools may even have affirmative action programs for chronically ill students. I don't really like to take handouts, but diabetes has made my life a little bit harder, and I have had to work harder to get where I am today, so I welcome anything that makes it a little bit easier.

I am fortunate that the university I attended, Stanford, offered all of these things. Some schools may not be able to offer these benefits because of limited resources, so be sure to look into what is available when you're making decisions. Letting as many offices and people at college know of my condition made the transition from living at home to living on my own as smooth as it was for everyone else.

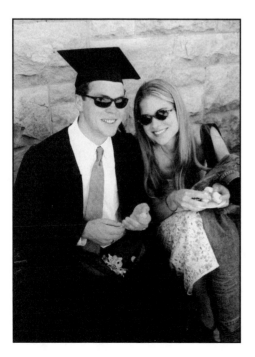

**Spike and Vanessa at Spike's Stanford graduation.**

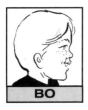

Our mom's book, *Real Life Parenting of Kids with Diabetes,* devotes a chapter to going off to college with lots of lists. This information will make your transition from home to dorm life a piece of cake.

# 12 Traveling the Globe on Your Own

## BACKPACKING THROUGH EUROPE

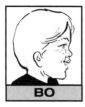
BO

Have you ever had someone tell you that you couldn't do something? When they told you this, what was the first thing you wanted to do? When I am told I can't do something, I always like to go out and prove my adversaries wrong. In high school one of my best friends, Ben, liked to scuba dive, so I figured I would learn how to scuba dive and get certified like Ben.

I grew up in a small town, and some way or another a local doctor heard that I was going to learn how to scuba dive. The next time I saw him he told me, "You should really be careful about scuba diving with your diabetes. It might not be a good idea." I immediately signed up for all the necessary scuba classes, passed the exams, and became a certified scuba diver. It felt great. Six weeks later I found myself having finished my last dive of the day and having a blast off Catalina Island with my friend Ben and his family.

What does this all mean? It means that you can do anything with your diabetes, whether it's scuba diving, driving, dating, traveling, or team sports—you just have to be organized in the way you approach it.

In the summer of 2004 I decided to backpack through Europe to prove to myself I could do it. I was going to be on my own, in foreign countries where I didn't know anyone, didn't speak the language, and didn't know where I was going or what I was going to do. I was going to be totally independent.

It's true, I was totally independent while I was in Europe, but I planned very well and took many extra precautions. The easiest part of my trip to Europe was deciding that I wanted to go. The hardest part was convincing my parents that everything would be OK. I had to plan, and plan well. I was going to backpack through Europe. The first thing was to figure out which countries I wanted to go to and how long I was going to be there. I planned on being gone for eight weeks. (I actually ended up being in Europe for 11 weeks.) Next, I started to think about what I needed to pack, particularly my diabetes and insulin supplies.

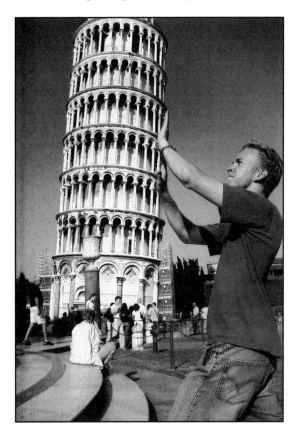

**Bo and the Leaning Tower of Pisa.**

# WHAT TO PACK

**Insulin** I needed eight weeks' worth of insulin, but I left room for error. I thought that if I was going to be traveling with just a backpack, chances are I might break one bottle, lose another, and one might get too hot in the sun and go bad. Knowing that I had to account for the unexpected, I decided to take double the amount of insulin that I would normally need. If I was using two bottles of insulin a month, I took four bottles for each month I planned on being in Europe, plus an extra two bottles in case I ended up staying longer than I originally planned (which turned out to be a good idea). I ended up packing ten bottles of insulin for an eight-week trip that ended up being an 11-week trip.

**Infusion Sites and Reservoirs** The same rule I used for my insulin applied to my infusion sites. I figured that I needed one infusion site and reservoir for every three days, but I needed to account for "error." Error in this case could be that I had to change an infusion site early because it was uncomfortable or that I went swimming, scuba diving, or surfing and my site fell off. Just like with the insulin, I took twice as many infusion sites and reservoirs as necessary. Here is how I figured out how many infusion sets to take: I planned on being in Europe for eight weeks. I would need to change my infusion site and a reservoir every three days. I would need: (8 weeks = 56 days, which is approximately 60 days). Sixty days divided by one infusion site and reservoir every three days equals twenty infusion sites and reservoirs. Remember, as a safety precaution I planned to take twice as many as I would need, so I packed forty infusion sites and reservoirs.

There are a few interesting things to note about diabetes supplies in Europe. Some cities in Europe do not have Humalog insulin. So this is what I did: I bought an international calling card and stayed up really late in California, where we are on Pacific Time. I called pharmacies in the major cities I planned to visit and asked what diabetes supplies they carried.

Even if pharmacies have a lot of diabetes supplies, they still don't sell insulin pump products. The only place to get Medtronic Mini-Med pump supplies is through Medtronic MiniMed. Granted, they will ship your supplies wherever you like. But, unlike syringes, you cannot just go buy pump supplies from a pharmacy.

**Spare Insulin Pump** If you are going to travel out of the country for any length of time, you can get a spare insulin pump, and it is really easy to do. Medtronic MiniMed makes my insulin pump. They have a "loaner pump" program where they will loan you a spare pump to take on vacation—in case their original insulin pump has a problem. About two months before I left for Europe I called the toll-free number on the back of my insulin pump, as if I were ordering supplies, and they connected me with the right department, and I arranged for a loaner pump to be sent to me.

**Syringes** Since I have been on the pump I have rarely used syringes, but I still always keep them around. The same is true when you travel. You never know when your pump may have a problem. If you get really high blood sugar and you don't trust your pump or your current infusion site, take an injection. If your battery dies, take an injection. If your pump malfunctions, take an injection. If you go scuba diving and can't wear your pump for a few hours, take multiple injections. There are lots of reasons to have syringes with you. Instead of remembering all the reasons why, just know that you should always have syringes with you.

**Test Strips** Virtually every pharmacy, even the really small ones in the small towns in Europe, had test strips for sale. But I have been to numerous pharmacies, even in the United States, where my particular brand of test strips are not sold.

Worst-case scenario: If you run out of test strips and you go into a pharmacy that doesn't sell your brand, you can always purchase a new testing device that uses the test strips that they sell. That can be expensive. Just plan ahead and take enough test strips to last the entire trip, but plan well. You will need to take into account that you might lose some test strips. You may even lose an entire bag. Have a backup plan in case some of your stuff is stolen. Pack some insulin, test strips, and infusion sites in a separate place.

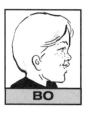

BO

Most of my supplies were in my main backpack, but I also had some in a smaller bag that I always kept on my person.

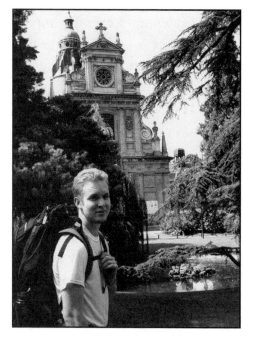

**Bo backpacking through Europe.**

**Lancets** It may be recommended that you change your lancet every time you test your blood sugar. (I do not change my lancet every time I test.) Figure out how often you like to change your lancet and make sure you take enough lancets to last. Be sure to take extra just in case.

## Contact Information

* **Pharmacies.** Plan well and do your research. Locate pharmacies all along your planned route and find out how you can get supplies from them if you need to.
* **Insulin Pump.** Bring your insulin pump manufacturer's international contact information.
* **International Telephone Numbers.** Medtronic MiniMed has international numbers that are easier to call while traveling in Europe. Get this information just in case you need it.

**Translations of Important Terms and Phrases** I can't tell you how important it is to be able to communicate a few important phrases, regardless of where you are or what language you are trying to speak. For my trip, I though I might need English, Spanish, French, Italian, German, Czech, Polish, Russian, Finnish, Turkish, and Arabic. The list might be a little long, but when you really need to be understood, having a few phrases printed on a piece of paper that you can hand to someone makes communicating very simple. I had a page for each language. Even though I speak Spanish and can communicate in Italian, I still had the key phrases written out. Who knows, I might get really low blood sugar and need to tell someone I have diabetes and I need sugar. It is easier to hand a waiter or a hotel concierge a piece of paper with the words "I have diabetes, I need sugar" written in Spanish than it would be to try to speak a foreign language when you have low blood sugar.

**BO**

Having these phrases about your health and your diabetes already printed out leaves no doubt in the mind of the person you are asking for help that you are serious and that you need help.

The easiest way I found to get all of the phrases translated was to go to my friends who speak these different languages and ask them to translate for me. When I couldn't find a friend to translate a particular language, I used an online translation program to translate my English phrases into a different language. You might also try *The Diabetes Travel Guide*, published by the American Diabetes Association, which provides translations of diabetes-related phrases in eight languages.

The following phrases are a must:

## Diabetes phrases
I have diabetes.
I need sugar.
I need insulin.
Can you help me find a pharmacy?
I need to eat.
I have low blood sugar.
I have high blood sugar.
This is my insulin pump.

## Non-diabetes phrases
How much does this cost?
Where is the restroom?
Thank you.
You are welcome.
You are beautiful (handsome).
You are very nice.
Thank you for your help.
Where is a nearby restaurant?
What is fun to do around here?

I can't tell you how many times I would frustrate someone by asking them a question in their language, a question I had practiced a number of times, and then not understand their response. Whenever this happened I always found it helpful to be really nice to them and compliment them. I was amazed at how helpful people became after I complimented them.

I took one backpack to Europe for an eight-week trip that turned into an 11-week trip. By the time I had packed all of my medical supplies, my backpack was more than three-fourths full. To the top of my backpack I added a box of granola bars, a pair of flip-flops, a pair of board shorts, a digital camera, a spare shirt, socks and boxers, and a thin raincoat. I wore my jeans, shoes, a shirt, and a warm jacket on the plane, and that was it.

Spike likes to say that having diabetes just means you have to be a little smarter and a little more organized. I agree with Spike and think he is right on the money, but the way I choose to look at it is that having diabetes is a gift that innately makes us a little smarter, a little more organized—and better looking, too.

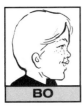 I am convinced that kids with diabetes live happier lives and make more money than their counterparts who don't have our gift. Think about it. If you have lived with diabetes, or have a close friend or relative with diabetes, then you already know how to manage a diet, blood glucose levels, exercise, insulin intake, insulin pumps, and all the other things that go along with it. By the time someone has lived with diabetes for two or three years they are chairman, president, and CEO of their health. This means that a seven-year-old may very well be the chairman, president, and CEO of his own company, Health Incorporated, by the time he is ten. How many other ten-year-olds do you know who are the presidents of their own companies?

## WHAT THE DOC SAYS:

Here is a master list of what to pack when you are going to be traveling in a foreign country:

### Diabetes Supplies

insulin
insulin pump and spare pump
infusion sites
reservoirs
batteries for the pump
syringes
glucose meter
test strips
lancets
ketone strips
glucagon shot (with directions on how to use it)
granola bars

### Non-Diabetes Supplies

passport
photocopy of your passport to be left at home in
  case you lose yours
phone card
debit card
credit card
$200 cash—small bills
camera (with the biggest memory card you can get)
jacket for everyday use
rain jacket
money belt
comfortable shoes
contact list of friends from home (send postcards)
contact list of pharmacies, friends, and relatives in the
  countries you will be visiting
sheet of terms and phrases translated into all the
  necessary languages

# 13 Insulin

## TWO KINDS OF INSULIN—ONE SYRINGE

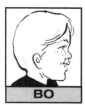 When you get used to using insulin three, four, or five times a day, you can forget what you have just done, so having a routine is important. Not as many kids are on NPH as there used to be, but if you are using insulins that the doctor tells you not **BO** to mix, following these steps will help avoid accidents and make your life a little easier. This is the routine Spike and I follow. When it is time for an injection, this is what I do:

Take two bottles of insulin out of the fridge and put them on the kitchen counter. I work from left to right, so I always put the Regular insulin on the left. I put the NPH insulin on the right. Then I double-check the bottles to make sure they are two different kinds of insulin.

I always draw the Regular (short-acting) first, which is the smaller amount. Then I follow by drawing the NPH.

## TWO KINDS OF INSULIN—TWO SYRINGES

In our teen years, we changed from NPH intermediate-acting insulin to Ultralente. Ultralente cannot be mixed with Regular insulin. A lot of kids use Lantus for their long-lasting insulin and, like Ultralente, Lantus cannot be mixed with Regular. With two bottles and two shots, you can get mixed up. To avoid using the same bottle twice (which equals a bad overdose, if it's two shots of Regular), we came up with the following system.

* Take two bottles of insulin out of the fridge. Put them on the kitchen counter— Regular on the left, Ultralente on the right.
* Put a needle in each bottle. Just leave them there sticking out.
* Draw the needed amount of Regular and inject.
* The second injection of insulin will be from the other bottle. The syringe is still in the bottle of Ultralente, so there is no mistake about which one to use.

We figured out this system after a couple of accidental overdoses. If you should inject with two doses of Regular or Humalog insulin, call your doctor immediately. Tell your mom and dad. You will need help getting through the next eight hours, but you can do it. Both Spike and I have accidentally overdosed on Regular. For the next eight hours, we tested every half hour, and we ate huge amounts of high-calorie food (Gatorade, candy bars, ice cream, bread—whatever we felt like).

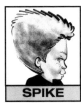

**SPIKE**

After an accidental overdose of insulin a glucagon injection is another option. You still need to tell your team what happened and get their help.

Doctors prescribe different combinations of insulin. You might be taking rapid-acting Humalog or Novolog and intermediate-acting NPH, or short-acting Regular and intermediate-acting NPH, or short-acting Regular and long-acting Lantus or Ultralente. Whatever the combination you use, the rules are the same.

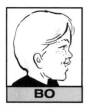

**BO**

Spike and I let our mom and dad draw the insulin and give the injections until we were teenagers. It was nice for us not to have to take on complete responsibility until we wanted to.

## WHAT THE DOC SAYS:

Although new kinds of insulin and new modes and schemes of insulin delivery may make things seem more complicated than they used to be, they actually give you more choices and flexibility than ever before. The basic goal of all insulin therapy is to deliver insulin in such a way that it balances calorie intake most of the time, giving you as close to normal blood sugars as possible. You will need to work closely with your diabetes educator, dietitian, and doctor to get the knowledge you need to empower you to take care of your diabetes best on a day-to-day basis.

# 14 Going on the Pump

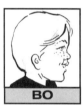

**BO**

When Spike and I first wrote Getting a Grip we were on injections. Then, in 2002, we both went on the pump. With the help of our friends, Julia, Mary, and little Laura, we'd like to tell you what it was like. (For a detailed account of going on the pump, see "The Adventures of Going on the Pump" in our book, *487 Really Cool Tips for Kids with Diabetes.*) When we made the switch from taking shots to using insulin pumps, we discovered many good things about switching—great things—and some trickier things that take a little getting used to.

## GETTING STARTED

Two weeks before going on the pump, Julia, Mary, and Laura worked with their diabetes educators, who showed them videos on pumping, taught them how to count carbs, answered all of their questions, and explained step-by-step how to use the pump. Spike and I had a similar lesson, but since we switched when we were a lot older, we took the quick one-day course. Like the girls, we were a little nervous about making such a big change, but our doctors and diabetes educators were able to answer all of our questions—including the ones we didn't know we had.

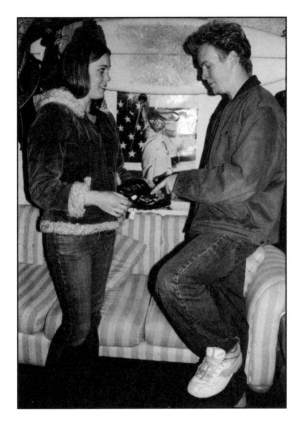

Mary Costello
and Bo,
looking at
Mary's pump.

A nurse helped the girls get fitted with their pumps. This is how you do it: You inject a small, short needle that has a tiny cannula (a soft, plastic tube) inside of it into your stomach near your belly button. Then you pull the needle out, leaving the cannula under the skin. An adhesive connection about the size of a quarter sticks right to your skin with a little piece of plastic that's about the size of an insulin bottle cap (called the "infusion site"). You plug the pump tubing into that. A very thin tube about thirty inches long goes from the connection to your pump.

After a few days of practicing pumping with saline solution, the girls filled the vials that sit in the pager-sized pump with Humalog and they were officially pumping! For the first few weeks they took lots of blood tests every few hours so they and their doctors could figure out what their "baseline" was. By testing very often and knowing exactly how much they were eating and how much insulin they were taking, they could figure out how much insulin they should have pumping into their body all day long. The pump injects a tiny bit of insulin, called the "basal," almost nonstop. When Spike and I first started pumping, our basal rates were about one unit of Humalog per hour. No one wants to take a shot every hour, but on a pump you don't have to—the insulin leaks into your body automatically.

Another great part about the pump is that instead of taking another shot every time you eat, you just test, count how many carbs you are planning on eating, and punch in how much insulin you need to cover the carbs. Voilà! The insulin gets delivered! Plus, you only have to switch your pump around once every three days, and that's it. For Spike, who was taking six shots a day before switching over, that meant going from 18 shots (pokes) in three days to just one poke—injecting the cannula—every three days.

As the girls have found out, one of the best parts about going on the pump is better control over their sugars. Sometimes, when I used to test and I was just a little bit higher than I wanted to be, I would wait an hour, until I was going to eat, to take any insulin. I didn't want to take a shot with just half a unit or so. Now, on the pump, if I test at 130 and want to be at 115, I just punch a few buttons and take a half unit—no shot, no problem! Pumping really makes it easier to "fine tune" your control. Spike and I had good control before we switched, and now it is even easier to have great control!

Of course, the pump does take a little getting used to. After all, you have a little tube sticking out of your side that wasn't there when you were taking shots.

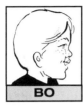

**BO**

I like to think of myself as kind of a bionic man now. Spike couldn't figure out how to reconnect the pump to the infusion site after taking it off to surf or shower. It is really easy; it is just that, for Spike, nothing even a little bit mechanical is ever easy!

Since we are no longer taking intermediate- and long-lasting insulin like NPH, Lantus, or Ultralente, we can't stay disconnected for too long, so when we are surfing or playing sports we have to paddle in or take a break and plug back in to our pumps to get some insulin back in our systems pretty frequently.

## SAFETY TIPS

✳ On field trips or camping trips, carry extra insulin and syringes, just in case your pump malfunctions.

✳ Carry extra triple A (AAA) batteries in case your batteries die while you are on a trip. You usually have to replace the batteries once a month or so, and the pump gives you a warning when the battery is getting low.

✳ It is always a good idea to have some syringes stashed in your car or backpack in case something happens with your pump.

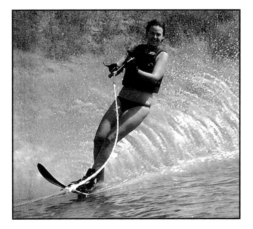

**Julia Halprin Jackson waterskiing and pumping!**

* You can always use the vial from the pump to get insulin if you have to take a few shots with a syringe until you fix your pump. (Disconnect your pump before drawing insulin with a syringe.)
* If you plan on taking a vacation to another country you can arrange to get a second "loaner pump" from your pump provider, just in case your pump breaks down.

## WHAT THE DOC SAYS:

When you want to keep your blood sugar levels closer to normal, you get into what is called intensive diabetes management. It's a three-part approach: nutrition, insulin, and exercise. You use carb counting or meal planning so that you can predict the effect the food you eat will have on your blood sugar and insulin needs. You use multiple daily injections of insulin or the pump to mimic the way your body provides insulin throughout the day to lower blood sugar. The pump supplies a basal amount of insulin slowly and evenly throughout the day and a bolus amount of insulin whenever you eat food. Exercise helps keep your body fit and improves the way your muscles use blood sugar.

You will need to check your blood sugar more often to learn how it reacts to different foods, insulin levels, and levels of exercise. You keep a written log of the foods you eat, the insulin you take, the exercise you get, the stress you're under, and your blood sugar levels. This helps you figure out your own patterns, so you can make decisions and changes in your self-care plan.

Some of the advantages of an intensive care plan:
1. You can keep your blood sugar closer to normal, so you feel better.
2. You give yourself the best chance for avoiding problems later in life.

> 3. You have more flexibility about when you eat and how much you eat.
>
> 4. You may improve your health and fitness level.
>
> **Some of the difficulties of an intensive care plan:**
>
> 1. You'll need detailed diabetes education.
>
> 2. You increase your risk of having hypoglycemia.
>
> 3. You may need motivation to keep doing all you have to do.
>
> 4. You'll increase the cost of maintaining your diabetes, with supplies and office visits.
>
> Intensive regimens are flexible because they get you out of the "two shots a day, have to eat right now!" mentality of diabetes care. If you are interested in trying out the flexible regimen, talk with your doctor or diabetes educator.

It is always interesting to see how Spike and I approach problems. Now that we are older we have a few more stories to share.

## THE USC ROSE BOWL GAME: THE DAY MY INSULIN PUMP BROKE

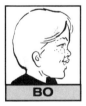

BO

It's 6:00 a.m.—yes, I woke up at 6:00 a.m. even though I do not have to work—and I am getting ready to change my insulin pump. When I change my pump site I often take a shower after I remove my old infusion site and before I put on my new site, so I can get all that sticky residue off. This morning is unlike most mornings, and it's not just because I woke up at 6:00 a.m. No, this morning is special on a much grander scale: my college football team, USC, is playing in the national championship

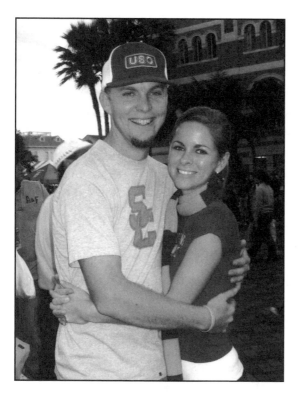

**Bo and Tami
at a USC
football game.**

game, and guess who got tickets? Good guess—but actually my girlfriend got the tickets and decided to take me with her!

After I remove my infusion site and take my shower, I get out a new reservoir and a new infusion site to get ready to put my pump back on. When I finish loading all the insulin into the reservoir, I do what I always do. I attach the infusion site to the reservoir and put the reservoir into the pump so that I can prime it.

By the way, when I say I am priming my pump, I am referring to the process that I go through to get my pump ready to wear each time I change my infusion site. Priming really amounts to getting the empty tubing that is part of the infusion site full of insulin. Just think about what would happen if you didn't put insulin in all that tubing (i.e., you didn't prime your pump). Then you would have hours of no insulin getting to your body because it would be filling the tubing. What does this mean? You must prime your pump every time you put in a new reservoir.

My brother and I always brag to one another about how little time we actually "have" diabetes each day. We add up how long it takes us to check our blood sugar and take our boluses, and whoever does it fastest wins. Yes, everything is competitive with us. Just so you know, I currently have diabetes for only four minutes a day, and my brother is stuck somewhere between four and a half and five minutes. Something that really adds time to my daily diabetes clock is having to change my infusion site, and today it ends up adding a lot of time to my clock.

So I have the reservoir in the insulin pump, and I begin to prime it. Usually when I do this the pump goes through a few phases. In the first phase the little screw on the pump extends until it hits the bottom of the reservoir and lets you know by beeping a few times so that you can prime the rest of the pump. The second phase is when you push enough insulin out of the reservoir to fill the entire tube. My particular insulin pump lets me know how many units it takes to fill the tube. Mine usually takes between 12 and 18 units of insulin to fill the tubing. The number of units it takes to fill the pump can change with the length of the tubing and with how much insulin you put in the reservoir.

So when did things start going wrong for me on this fine morning? I knew something wasn't right when I couldn't get my insulin pump to acknowledge that I was trying to prime it. I had the reservoir in the pump, and the "screw" that pushes the insulin out of the reservoir was extending. But instead of the pump sensing that the reservoir was in place, it pushed all the insulin out of the end of the tubing. That was when I knew something was wrong.

I try filling the reservoir with more insulin and priming it again. This does not work. I even try getting a new reservoir, thinking that the old one might be bad. That doesn't work either.

You know how I said I only have diabetes for about four minutes a day? Well, I'm ruining my average—I have now spent about twenty minutes trying to change my infusion site.

Realizing that it has been over half an hour since I received any insulin from my pump, I decide it would be a good idea to take some Humalog insulin the old-fashioned way. That's right, I get out a syringe. (Hmm, I think I bought these syringes about three years ago.) I test and take just one unit of Humalog to hold me for another thirty minutes.

After I play with my pump a little while longer, I realize that I am not going to be able to fix it. So I pick up the phone and call Medtronic MiniMed, the manufacturer, and explain my dilemma. The rep on the phone says that there is a sensor that sometimes malfunctions, and this particular sensor senses the pressure that the screw receives from the reservoir. In my case, my sensor may have been wiggled out of place and therefore does not know that the reservoir is in place. He asked me if my pump had been hit recently. Recalling all the times that I had played football, fallen while skateboarding, landed hard while skydiving, caught my tubing on a doorknob only to have my pump fly out of my pocket and crash against the door, or had just simply dropped my pump, I calmly tell him, no, I have not hit my pump recently. He is pretty convinced that the sensor is damaged and that I will have to get a replacement. I am convinced, too.

The rep says that I can have the pump shipped to me overnight or that I can pick it up from their warehouse. I tell him I will pick it up. Luckily, I'm not the only one in my family going to the Rose Bowl game. My parents, who are huge USC Trojan fans, are going as well, and they have to drive right past the MiniMed warehouse to get to the game.

For the next few hours, I inject at least one unit of Humalog insulin every hour in addition to any insulin I take for a meal

(meal bolus). I get my replacement pump from my parents at 2:30 p.m. This means I have taken about nine injections today—and all before dinner, too. On top of all the injections, I have tested my sugar a lot. I have not been on injections for years, and I know that without the insulin pump constantly giving me tiny doses of insulin my numbers aren't going to be as stable as normal. Sure enough, they aren't that great, but I never get low, and I never get too high, and things work out well.

Did you ever read Aesop's Fables? Well I did, and I liked the moral at the end of the story. The moral of this story: Having a plan for taking care of problems makes them into a minor inconvenience.

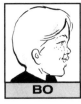 If you have problems with your insulin pump, disconnect it and go back to injections. Call the manufacturer of the pump and have them send you a replacement immediately. Test a lot and remember that you will need to either take long-acting insulin or take lots of shots of short-acting insulin. When I was on injections, one unit of rapid-acting insulin reduced my blood sugar by about 40 points. So I tested every hour, and I injected one unit of Humalog for every 40 points my blood sugar was over 120, as well as one unit of Humalog for every 13 carbohydrates I ate.

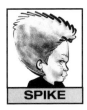 If your pump breaks and you need to go back to injecting insulin, you can use the insulin in the reservoir in your pump. Safety tip: Always remove your pump before sticking a syringe in the reservoir!

# THE USC VS. NOTRE DAME
# FOOTBALL GAME:
# THE DAY MY TUBING BROKE

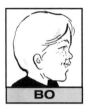

USC football isn't just a game; it's a way of life. So you shouldn't be surprised that I drove an hour and a half across town to watch a game with my girlfriend, Tami, and my closest buddies. Mind you, this was no ordinary game. This was one of the most storied rivalries in all of college football. The USC vs. Notre Dame game was arguably the biggest game in the college football regular season.

Tami picked me up and we headed to the store to get some food for the inevitable barbequing that would precede the kickoff. About thirty minutes before the scheduled kickoff time, I was walking through the TV room to get some more food. When I passed by the pool table, I felt something tug on my insulin pump. This sometimes happens when I walk by a doorknob or some other protruding object and the tubing on my insulin pump snags and tugs on my infusion site. But this time was different. When I looked down at my tubing I noticed that it was cut cleanly in half. No joke. My insulin tubing was literally cut in half!

What to do? Whenever something totally out of the ordinary like this happens, I always try to make a list in my head of what has happened and what needs to happen:

* I just broke the tubing of my insulin pump.
* I am no longer receiving insulin.
* I still have insulin left over in my reservoir.
* I need to get insulin into my body.
* I need to watch every second of the USC/Notre Dame football game.

Once I figured out what had happened and what that meant to me in terms of my insulin and my blood sugar levels, I immediately told my girlfriend Tami what was going on. It is not a good idea to keep something like this to yourself. Let everyone know what has happened, so if things don't work out as planned they can help.

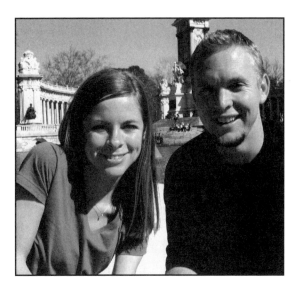

**Tami and Bo.**

Tami is a great girlfriend and very smart, and she happens to be studying health at USC. When I told her what was going on, she really helped me figure out what I needed to do. I knew that I had just bolused for a meal, and I checked to see that I had received my insulin. When I looked through my bolus history it showed that I had bolused about fifteen minutes ago, so I was pretty sure that I had gotten all of my insulin. I also noted that when I took my last bolus I had accounted for some chips and dip that I had not yet eaten. This was a good thing. This meant that, even though I was not currently receiving any insulin (my tubing was cut by this time), I had a little extra insulin in me. I decided to not eat the chips and dip so that the extra insulin could make up for the time that I was not going to have any insulin entering my body.

I needed to either go home to get a replacement infusion site with new tubing (I would normally have extra reservoirs and infusion sites and syringes and other diabetes supplies with me, but I was not driving my car today) or go to a pharmacy and get some syringes so that I could use the leftover insulin in my reservoir and give myself injections. Since we only had about thirty minutes until kickoff, I thought we'd better just go to a nearby pharmacy. Tami, being the caring girlfriend she is, wanted me to go home to get a replacement infusion set because, as she said, "I don't care about the football game as much as I care about you!" Yeah, she's a keeper. Being set on going to a pharmacy, I asked my buddy where the nearest one was. He told me that there was one within two blocks. Tami and I got over there, explained to the pharmacist what had happened, and got enough syringes to last the rest of the day.

Next came the tricky part. My pump wasn't going to be of any use to me, except for the insulin in the reservoir, so I was going to have to get my insulin by taking injections. This is how I approached it: I figured that I was getting about one unit every hour through my basal rate. So that would translate into an injection of about half a unit every half hour. I didn't want to go an entire hour between injections. I wanted to try to mimic the insulin pump by giving myself lots of injections of a little insulin.

By taking half a unit every half hour I had my basal rate covered, and I was testing my blood sugar a lot so if I got high I could take more insulin and if I got low I could eat more. By the end of the day, I had taken 12 injections—one every half hour for six hours to cover my basal rate. I also took a couple more insulin injections to account for meals and to correct for highs.

Here are some of the things I learned that day:

* If I had had all the supplies that I keep in my car I would have been able to use the long-acting insulin in my cooler, but since I didn't have any long-acting insulin I had to make do.
* When you run into trouble, let those around you know what happened, so they can help you if they need to.
* Know how to get to a pharmacy near you. You never know when you will forget supplies or have something unexpected happen.
* When it comes down to it, the two most important things are taking your insulin and monitoring your blood sugar. Regardless of the situation, if you can do those two things you will be OK.

## WHAT IS THIS CRACK IN MY PUMP?

SPIKE

I had an interesting adventure with my pump, too. Unlike Bo, technical guru that he is, it took me a long time to even figure out that my pump was acting funny.

I woke up pretty high several mornings in a row. By "pretty high" I mean anywhere from 220 to 320! I would instantly take a large correction bolus using my normal ratio of one unit for every 40 points of blood sugar. But instead of coming down to 120 or so, I would get super low super quick. By "super low" I mean 50 or even less. I had no idea why I was reacting so weirdly to my normal nighttime doses and my normal correction boluses. I should have called Bo because he tends to know about computers and toasters and pumps and things like that, but I just kind of went along like this—checking my blood sugar way more than normal—for three or four days, hoping I would start getting normal sugars.

After a few days of studying my pump I noticed something that wasn't there before. There was actually a little crack along the bottom—not big by any means, just sort of a little hairline crack. But it was getting bigger. I noticed that sometimes the crack would be pretty big, and I would push the bottom of my pump back together to make the crack hairline-thin again and then think nothing of it. A few hours later, the crack would be big yet again. "Well, that's weird," I thought, but since my sugars were still getting so low half the time, I figured I was still getting insulin and that my pump wasn't broken. That's what I get for thinking.

It turns out that every time the little screw in my pump turned and tried to push insulin into my body, it instead pushed the back end of my pump away, making the crack bigger. So the reservoir stayed just as full. At night, I wasn't getting any insulin. Then, in the morning, when I pushed my pump back together, the screw hit the reservoir and plunged a whole night's worth of insulin into me all at once—in addition to the extra units I took to come down from being so high! No wonder my sugars were so out of control—my pump was broken!

Now, I hate having my sugars all out of whack, and since I was sometimes overdosing by four or even five units, this was a pretty dangerous little episode. What made it worse was that all of this was going on just days before I had to take the LSAT (Law School Aptitude Test)—the test that would decide which law school I ended up at (basically, my fate) for the next three years. I did not want to go into this test not knowing if I was getting insulin and only knowing that my blood sugar was "somewhere between 50 and 350."

I called Medtronic MiniMed and they put a new pump in the mail right away. I went to my pharmacy for a fresh bottle of Ultralente. (I had some in my fridge, but it was close to two years past the expiration date.) I had to call my doc to get an updated prescription of Ultralente. Once I got home I just switched right back to my pre-pump routine. I took a shot of Ultralente to cover the next 12 hours, and I took shots of Humalog every time I ate or if my sugars were still high a few hours after meals. My sugars were not perfect, but they were way better than they had been with the broken pump.

The day of my big test the shiny new pump arrived from Medtronic MiniMed. I sent my old pump back in the same box they sent the new one in, waited until my 12-hour dose of Ultralente (from the night before) was out of my system, and went back to pumping. By the time I sat down that afternoon to take the test, I had my first consecutive blood tests between 90 and 120 for the whole week!

I learned a couple of lessons with this one:

* Your sugars normally won't go completely crazy for no reason whatsoever. I've had them out of whack from hormones (puberty), being sick, stress, bad insulin, and now a broken pump. When sugars are going nuts for a day or more, call your healthcare expert to help figure it out.
* When you have a problem with a pump, the manufacturers take it seriously and get you help as quick as possible. Medtronic MiniMed was super-awesome to deal with this so quickly.
* Even though all you use in a pump is short-acting insulin, it is a good idea to keep a prescription on file for long-lasting insulin like Lantus or Ultralente. If my doc had been on a golf trip, it could have been a much bigger hassle to get new Ultralente.
* Even though I felt pretty lousy the whole time my blood sugars were swinging so wildly, as soon as I figured out the prob-

lem and got a normal flow of insulin back, I felt great. I aced those LSATs only a few hours after I got a new pump plugged back in.

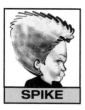

**SPIKE**

Any time I even suspect I am having a technical issue, whether it's with my VCR, my truck, or especially with my pump, I should call Bo.

# 15 Dealing with Doctors

Getting a good doctor or two is vital when you have diabetes. It is always good to have someone who really knows this stuff looking out for you. The twice-a-year major blood work visits are important, too. They can really tell your doctor a lot and help you to keep your blood sugar levels on target. However, one big thing with doctors is that they want what is absolutely the healthiest option for you, and this often conflicts with what you may want to do. There is generally a middle ground that will still keep you very healthy.

Some things to do to stay healthy:

* **Get a specialist.** Endocrinologists and others who specialize in the treatment of diabetes are a key to living healthy. They know things that no general practitioner would dream of, and they can often explain the processes of diabetes in understandable ways. Having an idea of what is going on in your body really helps you manage it. Besides, it's no fun to tell people "I don't know" when they ask you what diabetes really is.
* **Try to find a pediatrician or general practitioner with at least some background in diabetes.** Specialists are expensive and, chances are, you will only visit them a few times a year and only for diabetes-related issues and checkups. The doc-

tor who takes care of you all the rest of the time should know how different medications and ailments affect hormones and blood sugars. However, don't be afraid to call your specialist whenever you have any type of question.

✴ **Don't worry if you don't follow your doctor's orders exactly.** The doctor's advice is sound, and following it will keep you the healthiest but probably not the happiest. A piece of cake (a small piece) at a birthday party isn't bad. A day where you just sit on the couch (once in a while) is all right. Eating a little more when you are hungry is OK, too. Diabetes doesn't have to keep you from being a kid and having fun.

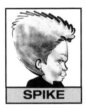

We had an ice cream party in my fifth grade class about a week after Bo and I had been in for a major checkup. I turned down all offers of ice cream and just sat outside and pitied myself. That is no way to live. It's perfectly fine to live it up a little and "cheat" a little (as long as it doesn't become a habit). I should have checked my blood sugar and taken enough insulin to counter-act a small bowl of ice cream and then eaten some. Don't mis-understand me here—it is extremely important to visit your specialist regularly and take what they have to say seriously. But it is also extremely important to enjoy your life.

## WHAT THE DOC SAYS:

I couldn't agree more! This topic brings up the issue of freedom versus responsibility. Remember: You can usually have both. I never use the word cheat when referring to a change in the ideal self-care plan. There is always a reason you don't follow your care plan to the letter, and it's important to look at it and recognize why, so you can make self-care decisions that serve you best. Don't be afraid to tell your doctor what is important to you. If you respect yourself and your desires and speak up, your doctor can usually find a way to work with you to keep your glucose on target in most situations. For example, most physicians no longer prohibit desserts but teach you how to incorporate them into your meal plan. Remember, it is your life you are talking about, and you are the expert on your life. At the same time, the knowledge and experience of diabetes professionals, parents, and other adults important in your life can also help you reach the goals you set for yourself. Your doctor and other diabetes care professionals are your expert consultants, and they are there to best serve your needs and interests.

# 16 When You Are Sick

Kids with diabetes get sick, too. If you are not feeling well, it's not always because of your blood sugar or because of your diabetes acting up. Still, it's not a bad idea to check your blood sugar and try to figure out what's going on. **Whenever you are feeling down, that's the first thing you should do—check your sugar.**

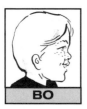

When you're sick, your blood sugar tends to run a little high. On top of being sick, high sugar makes you feel worse. Test your sugar often; you might need some extra short-acting insulin shots throughout the day. When I'm high, I take extra shots or boluses of two or three units of Humalog or Regular, drink lots of water, and check for ketones.

## SICK-DAY PLAN

Make sure your doctor OKs your sick-day regimen. Here's mine:

* **Nausea:** When you are nauseated, the rules change. Now there is the possibility of vomiting up your food, so you might want to drastically reduce the amount of insulin you take at any one time. Sometimes my doctor has me stop taking long-lasting

insulin for a day or two and take short-acting insulin every 4–6 hours. I drink lots of fluids with calories in them. For instance, when I get sick, I drink Gatorade and regular 7-Up and eat plain white toast. I also like to have Popsicles around because they are good and easy to eat. It's not usually a good idea to eat sugar, but when you're nauseated, you need the calories.

* **Vomiting:** If you vomit more than once, it's time to call your doctor. You'll need a prescription drug for the nausea. (We have a prescription for Compazine we keep at home and take with us when we travel. Note: Compazine is not used for children; choose Phenergan or Tigan.) You will need help. Your mom or dad should always stay home with you when you are nauseous or vomiting!

* **Compazine:** Knocks you out. Somebody must be home with you when you use it.

* **TLC:** When you are sick, you need attention. You need somebody to help you with all the blood testing and drinking. You need to keep your mind busy by watching TV or playing video games or using the computer. A back rub is always nice.

When you're sick, you'll probably be talking with your doctor. Don't get bummed out. Just remember, you'll get over it.

### Supplies to Keep on Hand for Sick Days

| | | |
|---|---|---|
| Regular 7-Up | Gatorade | Frosting |
| Sugar Popsicles | Plain white bread | Suckers |
| Chicken soup | Saltine crackers | Candy |

Liquids in very small amounts go down the best, and then I add Saltines and white bread.

Illness often makes your blood sugars go high, because the stress of illness causes the release of hormones (epinephrine, cortisol, glucagon, and growth hormone) that raise your blood sugar levels. On the other hand, if you are vomiting or you don't feel like eating much, your sugar may drop, and you will get low. It is important to always take insulin, even if you are vomiting and not eating. You may take only half your usual dose of long-acting insulin and take your short-acting insulin only after you see how much food you can keep down. Before you get sick, it is wise to set up a plan with your doctor for what to do. When you are sick, you should check your urine for ketones and take extra insulin as needed. If you are vomiting, check your blood sugar and urine ketones, and then call your doctor immediately.

## KETONES

When do you develop ketones? Sometimes, when you have had high blood sugar for several hours, you feel sick all over. Your body is achy, you feel sluggish—and you may have developed ketones. You should always have ketone strips around the house. Test for ketones when you're sick or when your blood sugar is running high. It's a simple urine test. This is how we handle ketones:

* **Ketone sticks.** After you dip the ketone stick in your urine, in a matter of seconds the stick turns colors. If dark purple shows up, you are making lots of ketones. Don't panic. You can get rid of ketones in a few hours. When I see high ketones on a ketone strip, I take a couple of extra units of Regular or Huma-

log insulin and drink a lot of water. I test for ketones every hour, watching the color on the strip fade until I'm back to normal.

* **Getting rid of ketones.** Spike and I look at testing for ketones as a positive thing. It's just another way to help you keep your blood sugars near normal. Lots of ketones means your body is burning fat and you may have had high blood sugar for several hours. When ketones show up, we work on getting rid of them right away. The first time you have high ketones you'll probably call your doctor. After that you'll know what to do: test, take a couple of extra units of short-acting insulin, eat a bite of food, relax, and drink lots of water. (We always eat a little when we inject insulin.) After an hour passes, test, and if ketones are still high, inject again and drink some more. Keep doing this until the ketones are gone. It may take only one session but sometimes it takes three or four. We never take more than two extra units of short-acting insulin late at night. We don't want to crash. (Crash is what we call what happens when your blood sugar gets really low, and you feel shaky, weak, and maybe emotional.)

* **Ketones and pumping.** When you are on the pump and you get ketones, you may need to take an injection of insulin with a syringe and change your infusion site. (If you are not sure your pump is delivering insulin, an injection with a syringe guarantees delivery!)

* **Ketones and vomiting.** If you are sick and vomiting and have ketones, it's time to call the doctor!

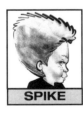
SPIKE

Ketones are tricky and can sneak up on you fast! If they aren't dealt with pretty quickly, they can make you real sick real fast. If I do a pee test and my ketones are high and I can't get them to at least come down a little over half a day or so, I always get help. I get help from my doctor, my parents, or even by checking myself in to the ER. There's nothing wrong with asking for help dealing with this stuff once in a while.

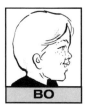
Remember the rule: Vomit once—call someone. Vomit twice—get help! The combination of ketones and vomiting can get serious fast! If you have ketones and you are vomiting, call your mom, dad, or doctor and get help!

## VOMITING

Vomiting is something that should always be taken very seriously. Whether it is the flu, food poisoning, ketones, or drinking too much alcohol that causes you to throw up, you need to be very careful. The general rule we live by is that if you throw up once, you call your parents, and if you throw up twice, you get help.

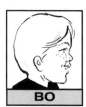
I got food poisoning recently and was the sickest I have ever been in my life. To add a complication to it all, when I got food poisoning my girlfriend was studying abroad in Spain and my roommate was out of town. Basically, my network of people closest to me was not available.

What happened was this: I went out to a nice dinner and enjoyed what I had to eat. After dinner I felt fine, and I went home to finish some work. As I was getting ready to go to bed, my stomach felt funny, but I thought nothing of it. The next morning I had no appetite for breakfast, which is strange for me, so I skipped breakfast and just had a glass of Gatorade. I made sure to take less insulin than normal. My stomach felt worse and worse all day, and I was not in the mood to eat, but I continued to sip Gatorade to get some calories in me just so I could function. By lunchtime, even the Gatorade wasn't settling well, so I walked to the nearby grocery store and bought some regular 7-Up.

I never drink regular sodas, but when you are having trouble eating, sometimes you just need to get calories however you can. If sipping on a regular clear soda was going to help me get some calories, then so be it. In total, my lunch consisted of about 2 ounces of regular 7-Up.

By the time 2:00 p.m. came around, I had already contacted my co-workers and told them that I wasn't feeling well and that I might need to take the rest of the day off. At this point I didn't know how true that would be. Within about twenty minutes of my phone call to my co-workers I found myself in the bathroom vomiting. My first session lasted a long time. I was vomiting consistently for about thirty minutes. I've had the flu before, and I have puked before. Even though I am an independent young man who can take care of himself, I knew that this time was different.

I couldn't get the rule about vomiting out of my mind: vomit once—call parents; vomit twice—get help. Since I had just finished my first of what would turn out to be many, many puking sessions, I called my parents to let them know that I was not feeling well and that I had just vomited. In the middle of the phone call I had to put down the phone because I started throwing up again. If it wasn't already clear, this second session made it obvious: I couldn't be alone that night. The next time I caught my breath I called my parents; they were already in their car on their way to pick me up and take me home.

For the next three days I battled food poisoning and dehydration. I couldn't keep any food down. In 48 hours the only "food" I had was half of one bottle of Gatorade. (I actually drank the entire bottle but threw up about half of it.) Needless to say, I wasn't getting many calories in my system and it showed. By the end of it all, I had lost nearly ten pounds, although most of it was water weight. But that food poisoning really took a toll on me. I ended up not making it to work on Monday, so that I could concentrate on re-hydrating and feeling better.

Here are some of the lessons I learned:

* **Take vomiting seriously.**
* **Getting dehydrated can make you really sick really fast.**
* **Diabetes is all about being organized and accounting for everything you do by taking insulin.** Normally, it's pretty easy. You take into account the food you eat, your blood sugar, and your exercise to help you figure out how much insulin to take. When you start vomiting, there is a lot more to account for, and managing your diabetes can become more difficult. That is why it is a good idea to have someone help you. And don't worry about needing help; it's a good thing!
* **I choose to look at asking for help as a way of empowering others.** People like to help others. It makes them feel good about themselves and inevitably builds stronger friendships, so don't be afraid to ask for help.
* **When you are vomiting, it is hard to tell how many calories you are actually absorbing.** When you start getting sick and dehydrated, lots of different hormones are racing around in your body, and they may affect your blood sugar and your sensitivity to insulin.

When you are sick:
* Test a lot, and when you take insulin, take it in small doses.
* Sip something with carbohydrates: Gatorade, regular 7-Up.
* Test more, and take lots of little doses of insulin.
* Always take your insulin after you have eaten, because you never know what your appetite will be, and you never know if

you will actually be able to keep the food down and absorb any of the calories.

✱ It's always safer to run a little high than it is to run low.

Make sure you have someone checking up on you. Have someone make sure you are up and awake at a specified time in the morning, say 8:00 a.m. Call your mom or dad. Have them phone you in the morning.

## WHAT THE DOC SAYS:

Ketones are acids that are produced when your body breaks down fat. If you have high blood sugar, too, ketones mean that you do not have enough insulin in your body to keep fat from breaking down. Your body gets rid of ketones in your urine, so it is important to drink lots of fluids if ketones are present. If ketones are produced more quickly than your kidneys can get rid of them, they will accumulate in your blood and cause nausea and vomiting. It is important to try to get rid of ketones before you get to this point, because nausea and vomiting can lead to dehydration and acidosis (too much acid in your blood). This can result in a vicious cycle in which vomiting leads to dehydration, which makes the ketoacidosis worse, which, in turn, causes more vomiting. At this point, you often need to be hospitalized and treated with intravenous (IV) fluids and insulin to break the cycle. The only way to keep ketones from forming is to take extra insulin.

Some people are very sensitive to insulin and only take small doses, but others are taking much larger doses. The dose of short-acting insulin that you will take to treat your ketones depends on your daily insulin dose. You should talk to your doctor or diabetes educator to determine the correct dose for you.

# GLUCAGON

Glucagon isn't just sugar as the name sounds. It is an anti-insulin hormone. That's why even when you can't eat any food, an injection of glucagon will raise your blood sugar immediately. Keep glucagon in your fridge or diabetes drawer, and always take your glucagon kit on trips.

## WHAT THE DOC SAYS:

Glucagon is a hormone that works like insulin in reverse. That is, insulin lowers blood sugar, and glucagon raises it. You need an up-to-date glucagon kit in your diabetes drawer or in the refrigerator—to be used by a family member or housemate—in case you have a severely low blood sugar and you are unable to take sugar by mouth on your own. Check now—if you don't have glucagon or your kit has expired, call your doctor's office for a new prescription. Everyone in the house needs to know when and how to use glucagon.

## When Do You Need Glucagon?

Your family members or roommates should inject you with glucagon if they can't wake you up or if you are so disoriented you don't make sense and they can't get you to eat.

## How Is Glucagon Injected?

1. Inject the liquid in the syringe into the bottle of glucagon powder.
2. Shake the bottle until the glucagon dissolves and becomes clear.
3. Draw all the glucagon solution into the syringe. (For kids who weigh less than 45 pounds, use half of the solution.)

4. Inject all the solution into the leg or butt.
5. Put the person getting the injection on his side, because he may throw up when he wakes up.
6. Give him food as soon as he wakes up: Gatorade, crackers, cookies, or anything he can eat.

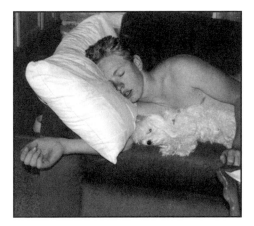

**Bo and Baby Dog taking it easy.**

# 17 Accidents or Surgery

## SPIKE'S SKATEBOARDING ADVENTURE

One morning while skateboarding to class, I had a little accident. Maneuvering through heavy student traffic, I hit a little bump in the road and my skateboard decided to stop. The only problem was that I kept going. I made a perfect landing on my left elbow, immediately picked myself up, and went on to class. Five days later I was in for orthopedic surgery.

When you go in for surgery, you never know exactly what's going to happen. For instance, the doc told me he was going to put a pair of pins in my arm and I would be out of surgery and back in my dorm room to study for finals in just a few short hours. As it turned out, the pins didn't work, so they went for the six-inch steel plate option and an operation that took about 4 1/2 hours and left me on morphine for three days. I was too doped up to take my finals, but I certainly learned a bit about dealing with diabetes while laid up in the hospital.

When you are going in for surgery:

* **Be in charge of your own insulin.** (You'll need your mom or dad helping on this job.)
* **Take your kits.** See pages 11–13.

* **Inform everyone you meet before, during, and after surgery that you have diabetes.**
* **Expect to use frequent small doses of insulin.** I took two units of short-acting insulin every few hours for the first two days. Pumpers: You'll want to decrease your basal a little, and you may not bolus much at all, depending on your sugars and meals.
* **Double check the doses when nurses are giving you your insulin.** (A cc is not the same as an insulin unit.) Many nurses are not used to the very small unit measurements on an insulin syringe. You must check what they want to give you every time. If you don't agree, discuss it. Ask questions! If pumping, you might have to train the nurses on how to operate your pump before the surgery even begins!

Better yet, take your mom or dad to surgery!

I'm going to outline what happened to me, so you will know what to expect if you have a snowboard or skateboard accident or other debilitating injury that requires surgery. Your doctor will be in charge, and the hospital will have a diabetes protocol. **Nevertheless, you are the one who knows the most about how to handle your own diabetes.** You're the expert on you.

* **The night before surgery:** I ate like a king—steak, baked potatoes, the works!
* **The morning of surgery:** No insulin, no food, no water.
* **During surgery:** My mother was there in the hospital, standing by. Have someone with you.
* **Post-surgery:** The recovery team did frequent blood sugar tests.
* **Post-surgery insulin:** The first insulin I received was three units of short-acting insulin at 3 p.m. that afternoon. I was groggy and then on morphine for two more days. My mom monitored my blood sugar and discussed every injection with the nursing staff.

We were surprised at how little insulin I needed to take those first two days. It made sense, though. I was eating almost nothing.

* **Nausea:** When coming out of the anesthesia, I needed something for nausea. Once the nausea was handled, I ate a little. Then it was determined how much insulin I should take. Again, it was only two or three units of short-acting insulin.

* **Post-surgery, day 2:** I had frequent blood sugar tests and frequent small doses of short-acting insulin. I didn't take any long-acting insulin until day 3. If you're on a pump, you can still take a basal; maybe just set it a lower rate than normal.

* **Post-surgery, day 3:** I returned to my dorm but was still on Vicodin, a heavy pain medication. We discovered that I was pretty out of it and needed help monitoring my diabetes, so I went home for a few days where my "support team" could take care of me.

In the hospital and post-surgery, you will need someone with you to help you handle your diabetes! I have always found that those closest to you want to be on your team. So go ahead and ask them for help.

## WHAT THE DOC SAYS:

The overall point here is a good one—nobody knows your body and diabetes better than you, and you should take an active role in your hospital management. However, situations such as those described here can be very complex. You will find it to your advantage to work with the members of your health care team in charge of your hospital care, since their medical knowledge will be most important to you at this stressful time. Balance is the key. While you don't want to get into power struggles with your hospital nurses or doctors over every insulin dose, you may at times need to assert that you are the expert on you, and they should respect your knowledge of your body and your diabetes.

# 18 Food— Short, Medium, and Long

When we were little, we made up this idea of putting all foods into the categories short, medium, and long. Short means that the sugar in the food gets into your system quickly. Medium foods take about 15 minutes to kick in, and long foods digest very slowly over a period of a couple of hours.

Here are some examples of each type:

* **Short:** All things with sugar, candy bars, granola bars, sugary cookies, milk, ice cream, cake with frosting, Gatorade, fruit juice, slushies, and smoothies are short. They contain sugar, which is a carbohydrate.
* **Medium:** Starchy things like bread, pasta, rice, chips, and crackers are medium. Starch is also a carbohydrate.
* **Long:** High-protein items like meat, chicken, fish, cheese, cottage cheese, eggs, and nuts are long.

## HANDY CATEGORIES

It's really handy to have food in these three categories. When you are little, it's a lot easier to understand "medium" than it is to understand carbohydrates. Since we had to eat every two hours (on our injection routine of combining Regular or Novolog with

NPH), we used short, medium, and long in our meal plans. As six-year-olds, we found it hard to remember that when you feel kind of down, you need a certain kind of food. It's easier to say, "I need a short," and somebody has it for you right there. Here are some other tips about short, medium, and long foods:

* **Friends:** When you are young and your folks tell your neighbors about your food needs, it's easier for them and your friends' parents to think about food as short, medium, and long.
* **Backpack:** Whenever you go anywhere, you need to have your backpack or your cooler with you packed with short, medium, and long foods.
* **Sports:** When you are about ready to play sports, it's OK to have a little short food.
* **TV:** When you're watching TV, you should snack on long foods and maybe a little medium.

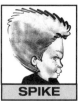

SPIKE

One of the great things about being on the pump is you don't have to snack as often!

Now that we are older and on the pump we have discovered that everybody who is on the pump counts carbs. (For a detailed account of carb counting, see *487 Really Cool Tips for Kids with Diabetes.*) When we first started counting carbs, we wrote down everything we ate and its carb count. Pretty soon we had our own handy carb-counting sheet.

All carbohydrates (short and medium foods) get converted to sugar. The body uses that sugar mainly for quick energy. Proteins and fats (long foods) are more slowly absorbed and don't act as quickly as carbohydrates. The carbohydrates that are most quickly absorbed act most rapidly on your blood sugar. These are the simple sugars found in fruit juices, hard candies, glucose tablets, and cake frosting (short foods). Other carbohydrates need to be digested and broken down to simple sugars before they can act. These carbohydrates include granola bars, cookies, cake, bread, pasta, rice, chips, and crackers (medium foods). When dealing with "short" or "medium" carbs, remember that everyone is different. For some people, some so-called medium carbs may act more like short carbs, so it's important to test these foods out for yourself to see how they work in your body. The more fat and protein a food contains, the more slowly it is absorbed and the more slowly it acts on your blood sugar. High-protein foods, such as meat, chicken, cheese, eggs, and nuts (long foods), are good for long-lasting endurance activities.

Spike and Bo have a good system for deciding what to eat and when. For example, if you are doing a high-intensity exercise for only a little while, then a medium food should work well for you.

Besides cake frosting, honey is useful for treating low blood sugar. There are glucose gels available, too, but you may not like the taste of them. Jerky is a long food that Spike and Bo like, but other people may prefer peanut butter crackers or half of a turkey sandwich. Any (long) food with protein and fat will help keep your blood sugar on an even level once you have raised it by eating a short food.

## SPIKE AND BO'S CARB-COUNTING SHEET

**Things we eat all the time**

| | | |
|---|---|---|
| Bagel—baby | 1 oz | 15 carbs* |
| Bagel—medium | 2 oz | 30 carbs* |
| Bagel—large | 4 oz | 60 carbs* |
| Banana | 1 small | 15 carbs |
| Beans, starchy | 1/2 cup | 15 carbs |
| Beer | 1 bottle (12 oz) | 13 carbs** |
| Lite beer | 1 bottle (12 oz) | 5 carbs** |
| Bread | 1 slice | 15 carbs |
| Brownie | 2-inch square | 15 carbs |
| Cereal, unsweetened | 3/4 cup | 15 carbs |
| Chips, potato | 13 | 15 carbs |
| Chips, tortilla | 13 | 15 carbs |
| Cottage cheese | 1 cup | 4 carbs |
| Crackers | 6 | 15 carbs |
| Cupcake, frosted | 1 | 30 carbs |
| English muffin | 1 | 30 carbs |
| Graham crackers | 3 squares | 15 carbs |
| Hamburger bun | 1 | 30 carbs |
| Hotdog bun | 1 | 30 carbs |
| Ice cream | 1/2 cup | 15 carbs |
| In-N-Out burger | 1 | 40 carbs |
| Double-Double | 1 | 40 carbs |
| Fries (McDonald's) | medium | 47 carbs |
| Macaroni | 1/3 cup | 15 carbs |
| Milk, whole | 1 cup (8 oz) | 12 carbs |
| Milk, whole | 12 oz | 18 carbs |
| Noodles | 1/3 cup | 15 carbs |
| Oatmeal | 1/2 cup | 15 carbs |
| Orange juice | 1/2 cup | 15 carbs |
| Peanut butter | 2 Tbsp | 7 carbs |
| Pie, pumpkin | 1/8 pie | 30 carbs |

## SPIKE AND BO'S CARB-COUNTING SHEET (cont.)

| | | |
|---|---|---|
| Popcorn | 3 cups | 15 carbs |
| Potato, baked | small | 30 carbs |
| Potato, mashed | 1/2 cup | 15 carbs |
| Rice | 1/3 cup | 15 carbs*** |
| Rice | 1 cup | 45 carbs |
| Spaghetti sauce | 1/2 cup | 15 carbs |
| Syrup, light | 2 Tbsp | 15 carbs |
| Syrup, regular | 1 Tbsp | 15 carbs |
| Tomato sauce | 1/2 cup | 5 carbs |
| Tortilla, corn | 6-inch | 15 carbs |
| Tortilla, flour | 6-inch | 15 carbs |
| Vanilla wafers | 5 | 15 carbs |

*Snack bars*

| | |
|---|---|
| Balance Gold–Caramel Nut Blast | 22 carbs |
| Extend Bar | 30 carbs |
|   Made with cornstarch for slow release | |
| Glucerna Bar | 24 carbs |
|   Made with cornstarch for slow release | |
| Granola Bar–Quaker Chewy Choc Chip | 21 carbs |
|   Always in our cooler | |
| Power Bar–Peanut butter 45 carbs | |

   * Bagels are dense and full of carbs—check the label.
  ** Beer can lower blood sugar. See beer, pages 67 and 69.
*** Notice that 1/3 cup of rice has 15 carbs.

Meat, chicken, salad, and vegetables are free unless you have a giant serving.

When you look at a label, only use the carb count. (Sugars are included in the total amount of carbs on the label.)

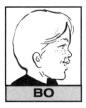

Check the back of packages for things you eat all the time. Then add your favorite foods to your personal carb sheet. We discovered that the flour tortillas we like have 20 grams of carb per tortilla.

## MEALS AND SNACKS WE LIKE TO EAT

Here is a list of some of the things we like to eat. We eat what we like; we just make sure we always have protein with carbohydrates. Our rule for meals and snacks: Never eat a carbohydrate alone.

### Breakfast

Every morning our mom makes breakfast. By far our favorite is the breakfast burrito.

**Breakfast Burrito (47 carbs)**

| | | |
|---|---|---|
| Flour tortilla | 10-inch | 20 carbs |
| Scrambled eggs | 1 or 2 eggs | |
| Sausage | 1 or 2 links | |
| Cheese, grated | small handful | |
| Fried potatoes | 1/2 cup | 15 carbs |
| Fresh salsa | | |
| Whole milk | 1 cup | 12 carbs |

**Another Sample Breakfast (42 carbs)**

| | | |
|---|---|---|
| Bacon | 1 or 2 strips | |
| Eggs | 1 or 2 eggs | |
| Potatoes | 1/2 cup | 15 carbs |
| Cheese, grated | small handful | |
| Toast | 1 slice | 15 carbs |
| Whole milk | 1 cup | 12 carbs |

We drink a glass of water with breakfast if we're high, a half glass of orange juice if we are low, or a half glass of whole milk if we're just right or starving. As you get older, you can increase the portions.

## Snacks

When we were little, we ate a snack every two hours. Kids using NPH must snack when the NPH kicks in (that's two hours after injecting). Every morning before school, our mom packed three separate snacks in three separate brown paper bags with the time written on each: 10 a.m. (snack), noon (lunch), and 2 p.m. (snack). The bag went into the top of our coolers. It was a tight squeeze, but it made snacking easy.

| 10 a.m. | Noon | 2 p.m. |
|---|---|---|
| String cheese | Trail mix | Crackers and cheese |
| Small banana | String cheese | Jerky |
| Crackers | Crackers | Grapes |

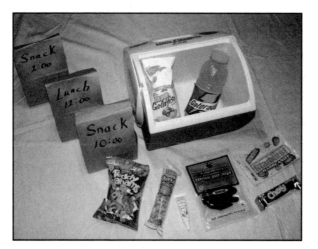

With rapid-acting insulin, many children and teenagers don't eat mid-morning snacks. It is important to determine your individual snack needs based on your insulin regimen and exercise programs.

## Lunch

Our favorite lunch is a breakfast burrito. Here are two other examples:

### Sample Lunch 1 (57 carbs)

| | | |
|---|---|---|
| BLT Sandwich | 2 slices bread | 30 carbs |
| Milk | 1 cup (8 oz) | 12 carbs |
| Small banana | | 15 carbs |

### Sample Lunch 2 (57 carbs)

| | | |
|---|---|---|
| Hot dog and bun | | 30 carbs |
| Small apple | | 15 carbs |
| Milk | 1 cup (8 oz) | 12 carbs |

I used to take my mom's famous breakfast burritos to school for lunch. My friends started noticing that I had them every day. They tried them, and they really liked them. Pretty soon I was taking extra burritos to school every day to share with my friends.

## Soccer Games

If we had a soccer game after school, Mom packed the following items in our athletic bags:

| | | |
|---|---|---|
| 1 box of crackers | 1 bag of beef jerky | 1 tube of frosting |
| 1 small box cookies | 1 large Gatorade | $5.00 |

## Dinner

When you have dinner, just combine your carbs with protein. If you are eating spaghetti, have a smaller helping of noodles with a big helping of meat sauce. When we are playing sports, we sometimes have spaghetti with a T-bone steak on the side.

Again, if we're high, we drink water with our meals. If we're low, we drink whole milk. Here are some examples of the dinners we eat:

**Sample Dinner 1 (57 carbs)**

| | | |
|---|---|---|
| Chicken | | |
| Potatoes, boiled | 1 cup | 30 carbs |
| Peas | 1/2 cup | 15 carbs |
| Milk | 1 cup (8 oz) | 12 carbs |

**Sample Dinner 2 (47 carbs)**

| | | |
|---|---|---|
| Tacos | 1 corn tortilla | 15 carbs |
| Beef, cheese, lettuce | | |
| Spanish rice | 1/2 cup | 20 carbs |
| Milk | 1 cup (8 oz) | 12 carbs |

## Bedtime Snack

Always eat a bedtime snack. Combine a medium and a long food (a carb and a protein). Here are some good examples:

| | | |
|---|---|---|
| Toast with peanut butter | 1 slice bread | 15 carbs |
| A second helping of dinner | | |
| Cereal with milk, plus either string cheese or peanuts | 1 cup cereal<br>1 cup milk | 15 carbs<br>12 carbs |
| A tortilla with melted cheese | 1 tortilla | 15 carbs |

Because we play sports, we tend to eat pretty large bedtime snacks. You won't need so much food right before bed if you have had a quiet day. Never skip a bedtime snack. (If you go to bed, are about to fall off to sleep, and then remember you forgot your snack, get up and snack. That way you'll have a good night and a good morning.)

## WHAT THE DOC SAYS:

When you're a teenager, eating well gives you the right amount of fuel, or calories, for normal growth and development and improves your overall health. In general, I recommend lots of fresh fruits and vegetables; whole grains; low-fat or fat-free milk; lean meats, poultry, and fish; healthy fats like nuts, avocado, and olive oil; and to the extent that your budget allows, organic foods free of pesticides and with no chemical processing. We all know that fast foods, high-fat sweets, and sugar-containing sodas taste good—I like to call them "play" foods. It makes common sense to eat these play foods only in moderation, because they give you very little nutritional benefit for all the calories they also give you.

Remember that even though there is no such thing as a "bad" or "forbidden" food, when you add sweets to your meal plan, it's important to trade them gram for gram for the other carbohydrates you would normally eat. That way, you're less likely to get high blood sugars or gain weight. Your dietitian can help you develop a meal plan to fit you and your lifestyle at the age you are right now. The meal plan will need to be changed as you grow, add sports or new activities, or want to try different foods.

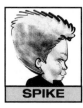
**SPIKE**

Pumping changes snacking. Once you get your nighttime basal rates adjusted, you won't always have to snack before bed. But after a day playing sports you will still need a bedtime snack.

## WHAT ARE PROTEINS AND CARBS?

Remember short, medium, and long? Each meal should contain protein, carbohydrates, fat, and vegetables. Here is a list of food to keep in the house, so you can have good stuff to eat without making your blood sugars go wild.

| Short | Medium | Long |
|---|---|---|
| Fruit juices | Beans | Beef |
| Hard candy | Cereal | Bacon |
| Milk | Crackers, chips | Chicken |
| Frosting in a tub in the fridge | Pasta | Cheese |
| | Potatoes | Cottage cheese |
| Frosting in tubes for emergencies | Rice | Eggs |
| | Whole fruits | Ham |
| Glucose tablets | | Hamburger |
| Gatorade | | Hot dogs |
| Orange juice | | Sausage |
| Regular 7-Up | | String cheese |
| Sugary cookies | | Fish |
| Cake with frosting | | Peanut butter |
| | | Turkey |
| | | Tuna |
| | | Jerky |

Always having these things on hand at home makes life simpler and more routine. The sugar drinks and frosting are for treating low blood sugar and should not to be eaten by anybody else. The frosting in the tub and regular 7-Up are for when you are really low.

All the kids in the family should know where the frosting is and should get it and give it to you immediately if you're feeling bad (one big spoonful).

Never put off eating when you have low blood sugar. Follow the frosting with whole milk. The sugar in the frosting will only last a few minutes. You'll need more long-lasting calories right away. Milk works great. Gatorade is also good if you catch yourself crashing. Crackers and cookies are a good second snack after a low blood sugar. Jerky just finishes off the snack, so you'll be in good shape.

## WHAT THE DOC SAYS:

For you science buffs, here's some extra detail you might find interesting. While both proteins and carbohydrates contain approximately 4 calories per gram, they serve very different purposes in our bodies. Proteins are for structure and action. For instance, the solid mass of our muscles is mainly protein, as are the enzymes needed for many important biochemical processes. Carbohydrates, on the other hand, primarily provide the energy our bodies need to function.

It is mostly the carbohydrate you eat that raises your blood sugar, so as far as blood sugar goes, the amount of carbs in the meal is the most important number. If you figure out how many grams of carbohydrate you eat in a meal, you can match it with the right amount of insulin to bring your blood sugar back to normal. Counting carbs offers you a huge amount of freedom and flexibility in your daily life, as you decide what to eat and adjust your insulin accordingly. If you need more information on carb counting and how it can benefit you, consult your registered dietitian (RD) or certified diabetes educator (CDE).

Finally, here are some important food and snack rules to keep in mind:

* Always try to eat some protein with carbohydrates.
* Fill the house with proteins for snacks.
* Have sugar foods around for when you are low.

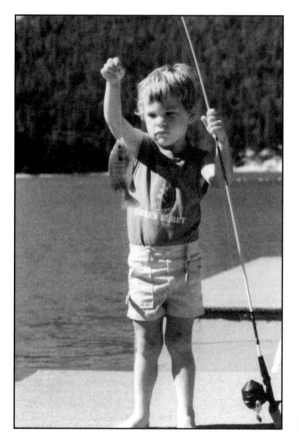

**Spike fishing.**

# 19 What Everyone Needs to Know— So They Can Help

This chapter contains three important documents: a list of symptoms of low blood sugar, an explanation of why kids with diabetes sometimes need extra calories, and a schedule of the things you do every day to take care of your diabetes. Your parents can copy the three documents in this chapter and substitute the important information about you. Give these documents to every teacher, principal, and coach you meet. Give a copy to your friends' parents, too.

## SYMPTOMS

Tape a copy of the symptoms page into the top of your cooler. This page tells people what symptoms to look for and gives clear directions for what needs to be done when you suffer a low blood sugar—when you crash. This is the document that works for us. Replace my name with yours and list your specific symptoms. Give this page to all teachers, coaches, parents, and close friends. Also make sure you have a "Permission to Treat" document on file at your local hospital and at your school.

## SYMPTOMS OF LOW BLOOD SUGAR

**Emergency Instructions for Helping Bo**

**When Bo shows these symptoms...**

| | |
|---|---|
| Mild: | Headache |
| | Stomachache |
| | |
| Serious: | Feels empty |
| | Shaky hands |
| | Feels faint |
| | |
| Extreme: | Very upset |
| | Crying |
| | Angry |

**Do this:**

1. Give fruit drink (Gatorade) from backpack.
2. Follow with granola bar, crackers, and then jerky. He should feel better in 3–5 minutes.

**Note:** These symptoms are listed in the order they usually appear. If you are with Bo while he is feeling empty and is shaky, crying, or upset, then you need to open the juice can or Gatorade, put it into his hands, and make sure he drinks it. Hand him the opened granola bar and make sure he eats it. These symptoms occur because his blood sugar is dangerously low. He is about to pass out. At this point his thinking is cloudy, he cannot function, and he needs sugar!

## SYMPTOMS OF LOW BLOOD SUGAR (cont.)

**Serious Emergency**

If you see the more serious symptoms after giving Bo a sugar drink:

1. Give him some more sugar drink. In about five minutes, follow with sugary cookies or milk (short), crackers or chips (medium), and jerky (long).
2. Then call Virginia (mom) or Rick (dad).

**Extreme Emergency**

If Bo should pass out:

1. Open frosting in backpack immediately. Squirt all of it into the corner of his mouth between cheek and gums. If no frosting is available, put sugar in the corner of his mouth between cheek and gums.
2. As soon as he is alert enough to swallow, follow with a fruit drink, real Coke, or Gatorade. Call Virginia or Rick. If no luck, call 911 or go to a hospital. Tell them he is suffering from low blood sugar, which is also called insulin shock, and he needs glucose.

Mom's phone numbers
Home: _____ Cell: _____ Work: _____

Dad's phone numbers
Home: _____ Cell: _____ Work: _____

Doctor's phone number:
Office:_____ Emergency number: _____

Hospital phone number: _____

# WHY KIDS WITH DIABETES OFTEN NEED EXTRA CALORIES

This explanation about why you need extra calories should come from your folks. It gives teachers and coaches an understanding of what is going on with your body and how they can help. This document explains why you eat so often. It's a lot easier when your teachers and coaches are aware of how often you need to eat. First of all, they won't hassle you, and second, they will be more supportive.

## WHY BO NEEDS TO EAT

Maintaining normal blood sugar in a growing kid who has diabetes requires an absolute constant flow of calories into the system. Bo must be allowed to eat the moment he senses that his blood sugar is low or dropping, in addition to eating his scheduled snacks.

Here are some things you need to know:

* **Eating:** Bo eats when he feels low. He also eats a snack every two hours. He needs more calories when he exercises and takes tests.
* **Behavior changes:** Bo doesn't always feel a low blood sugar coming on. If you notice odd behavior, ask him if he needs calories.
* **Vomiting:** If Bo vomits, he needs immediate calories, liquids, and care at home.
* **Injuries:** An injury can make blood sugar soar and then fall. If Bo gets injured, call Virginia (mom). She will come down and do some tests.
* **Blood tests:** Bo will need to do blood tests at school sometimes. All the kids know about these tests. Do not send Bo off alone for a blood test. He is probably test-

## WHY BO NEEDS TO EAT (cont.)

ing his blood because he is feeling low, and he may need some help to test and eat.

* **Calling home:** Bo needs to call home when he feels "funny" or bad. First have him snack. Then have a student walk to the office with him. Low blood sugar can cause him to become disoriented.
* **Understanding:** Teachers should not humiliate Bo about his calorie needs.
* **Vigilance:** Bo plays all-star soccer, surfs, and snowboards. He can do anything. We simply must be vigilant about his blood sugar levels EVERY TIME.

## WHAT THE DOC SAYS:

The important concept here is not so much the extra calories as it is the timing of the calories. A teenager with diabetes does not actually need any more calories than a teenager without diabetes, but he or she does need free access to food at all times in case of an unexpected low blood sugar. Unfortunately, this need can conflict with the rules and schedules of your school or other programs. It is very important that you talk about this special need with the people in charge to avoid unnecessary, frustrating, and possibly dangerous conflicts when you feel low between scheduled meals and need to eat a snack. The general principle appears in this book again and again—plan ahead so you can set up a situation around you that allows you the freedom you need to care for your diabetes.

# YOUR SCHEDULE

This page describes what you do every day. When adults get this schedule, it helps them understand you and diabetes. They can see on paper how hard you try to maintain normal blood sugars, so they tend to be helpful and understanding when you need to reschedule a test or are late for school.

| BO'S DIABETES CARE SCHEDULE | |
|---|---|
| 6:30 a.m. | Blood test<br>Insulin injection: Regular (short-acting) and NPH (intermediate-acting)<br>Breakfast |
| 8:30 a.m. | Snack—NPH kicks in |
| 10:30 a.m. | Snack |
| 12:30 p.m. | Blood test<br>Insulin injection: Regular<br>Lunch |
| 2:30 p.m. | Snack<br>Blood test |
| 4:30 p.m. | Snack |
| 6:30 p.m. | Blood test<br>Insulin injection: Regular<br>Dinner |
| 8:30 p.m. | Blood test<br>Insulin injection: NPH<br>Snack |

I work hard every day to balance what is going on in my body and to keep my blood sugars normal. Many things influence how insulin is absorbed and whether my blood sugar levels go up or down:

## BO'S DIABETES CARE SCHEDULE (cont.)

* **Exercise:** Lowers blood sugar rapidly. During soccer games, I snack every 15 minutes and do a blood sugar check at halftime.
* **Stress:** Usually lowers my blood sugar. During exams and heavy concentration, the brain absorbs enormous amounts of sugar. Blood sugar can drop dramatically, causing lapses in mental function. I just can't think. Eating a snack and taking 5–10 minutes to absorb the glucose gets me back on track.
* **Cold:** Lowers blood sugar rapidly.
* **Heat:** Changes insulin needs.
* **Illness:** Usually causes a rise in blood sugar. When I am ill, I usually take two or three additional shots of Regular (short-acting insulin) per day, check my blood sugar frequently, and test for ketones (acids that are produced when your body breaks down fat).
* **Growth spurts, hormones:** Usually cause a rise in blood sugar, which can make you feel "hyper." Very high blood sugar usually causes sluggishness and an all-over sick feeling.

## WHAT THE DOC SAYS:

Yet again, planning ahead, anticipating problems, and enlisting the understanding and support of the people around you are vitally important to provide the structure you need to be truly free and safe. There is nothing to be embarrassed about or ashamed of, so let all the adults or supervisors of your activities know your daily schedule. In fact, it can be a badge of pride to say, "I do everything I do in my life, and I do all this other stuff that most people don't have to!"

# 20 Brothers and Sisters

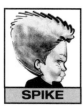
SPIKE

Diabetes has been a major part of my life and the rest of my family's since I was first diagnosed. We have all written various pieces about living with it, either for school assignments or just to get our feelings out. My brother, Bo, made a picture book when he was six, just months after being diagnosed with diabetes himself. It was hard for him to write about himself, so he chose to write about me. Every kid with diabetes should write about how diabetes makes him or her feel. It helps a lot. Even siblings who do not have diabetes can benefit from putting their feelings down on paper.

My sister Mary wrote the following essay during her senior year at Nordhoff High School. She entered a statewide essay contest to answer the question, "Should animals be used in medical research?" She won a $500 scholarship for her essay. Even siblings who do not have diabetes can benefit from putting their feelings down on paper. Mary went on to work for a research lab in San Diego, where she studied islets of Langerhans. She has now graduated from USC medical school and is in her residency at UCLA.

"Kids, I'm Proud of You" was written by my sister Jenny. Jenny is the oldest, and she was the boss when we were growing up. Don't let her four-foot-ten stature fool you; Jenny is tough. She received her B.A. from Berkeley in 1996 and is currently the editor-in-chief of *Kitchen Sink*, a San Francisco Bay Area culture and politics magazine. She is president of the Neighbor Lady Community Art Project, a nonprofit organization dedicated to arts and culture education.

The third piece in this chapter is an e-mail I wrote to Bo after my roommates at college had to call 911 for me. We figured out what happened and have included "911—One, Two, Three, Boom! You're Gone" to help you avoid the same situation. This story is not for little kids. When you go out on your own, you'll need to know how to handle every situation. We hope this will help.

## WHY ANIMALS ARE USED IN BIOMEDICAL RESEARCH

**by Mary Loy**

The experimental use of animals in medical and biological sciences is something I consider not only a very important part of science, but it is also something that is important to me personally. My reasons for my avid support of scientific research on animals will be apparent when you read about a painful but sobering scenario that took place in my home less than a year ago.

"Mom, I'm hungry."

"I know, honey, but you just ate."

"I'm so sick of this, Mom. I just want to be able to eat when I'm hungry like everybody else. Just give me a unit so I can eat."

A unit of insulin is what he meant. My brother is a diabetic. Diagnosed at age six, Thanksgiving Day of 1988, exactly one year after my other brother had been diagnosed at age seven. Hearing these words come out of my baby brother's mouth, it hit me. I suddenly realized that he had been unjustly and cruelly stripped of his innocence. He was right—he was no longer "like everybody else."

When we are hungry, we eat; it's part of our nature. When we are tired, we sleep in. When we want to play, we play. But my brothers can't just spontaneously do these things. They have to worry about what and when they eat, how and when they exercise, and how much insulin they need each morning and night, every day of their lives.

I'm a practical person. When Spike got diabetes, it was a shock for the whole family, and it was an awful thing to have happen. But I decided that it was a part of all of our lives now, and we would just have to learn to deal with it, however unpleasant or

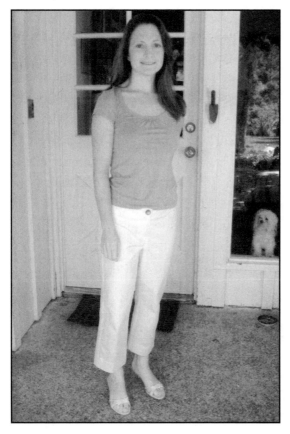

**Our sister, "Doc" Mary.**

unfair it seemed. When Bodie turned up with it, and we hadn't found any traces of the disease anywhere in our family background, I thought that if there is a God, he must be mad at our family. I couldn't understand how such a freak thing could have happened to us. But again, I was determined not to get emotional. At least they were both still alive, I told myself. At least with modern technology, they would both be able to lead almost perfectly normal lives. Almost.

So when I heard my brother utter that pitiful plea, "Just give me a unit so I can eat" with tears in his eyes, I wanted to take him into my arms and assure him that everything was going to be all right. But I couldn't, because it wasn't. My little brother I saw as this little hellion running around without a worry in the world, and I always felt I could protect him and say, "Don't worry, Bodie, I won't ever let anything bad happen to you." But he had been forced to grow up and become a responsible adult before most kids had learned to dress themselves. My image of him had changed; I no longer saw the same smiling, carefree kid. The smile was gone. I saw the eyes of an older man in my brother's eyes— one who had faced many hardships yet never found happiness.

Suddenly, all the problems I had considered to be such a big part of my life seemed insignificant and trivial. I was mad and frustrated. I couldn't protect little Bodie anymore; I couldn't undo what had already happened; I couldn't even take it away from him and put it in myself. I didn't want to be perfectly healthy while Bodie ("my little prince" is what my mother always called him) had to suffer.

This thing, this disease has changed him, I thought. He's so much more responsible; he's even a bit more sensitive. But he shouldn't have to be.

I console myself now with the knowledge that research involving experiments with dogs and swine is being done right now to try to find a cure for diabetes. This research is so exciting to me because it may mean that my brothers will be cured in the not too distant future. Having seen some of the experiments involving swine firsthand, I have been so inspired that I plan my own future in the field of medical research.

So many people can benefit from what science discovers through the use of animals in research, and so many wonderful and brilliant discoveries have already been made. I have chosen to focus on only one reason that this area of science is so important, simply because it is something that really hits home for me—and because I couldn't possibly cover everything that should be known about this marvelous field of study.

So when the question is asked, "Why are animals used in biomedical research?" My answer is, "Because of my brothers and others like them who can benefit from such research." If it can make a little boy's tears go away, nothing is more important.

## KIDS, I'M PROUD OF YOU

### by Jenny Loy

When Spike got diabetes, we all learned about how to be patient and help him when he was low and how to give shots. Even baby Bo, who was only five years old, knew where the frosting was and walked around the house practicing injecting an orange. Then Bo got diabetes, and we were really busy.

Mom was proud of us. "Kids, I'm proud of you, all of you." That's what she said one afternoon, herding us into the living room from the far corners of our after-school lives. Spike and Bo shuffled their feet a bit and the dirt from their latest war games sifted audibly to the floor. Mary and I stood behind the boys poking at them to watch the dust cloud slowly engulf their feet.

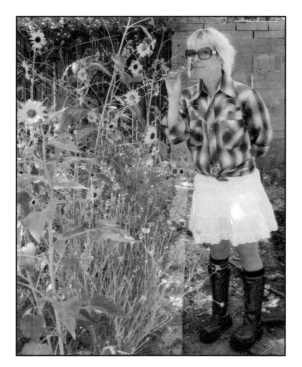

**Our sister, Jen, the writer.**

"Listen you guys, I'm really pleased with the way you've all worked together. You are like a little army taking care of each other. You've all been so wonderful." (You know how moms get.) "Your dad and I think you deserve a reward."

"Like what? A pack of gum?" I asked.

"No, a big reward," she came back. "You guys think of something you would really like to do, something big."

A huddle just wasn't going to be sufficient. Mary grabbed Bodie by the hand and I yanked Spike's collar. We hustled out of the living room so fast that the boys' GI Joe dust cloud was all that was left to hear Mom's hints. "You all like the ocean," she prattled away. "I was thinking of a trip to Hawaii this summer. I want to do something special for all of you."

We corralled the boys in the hallway where we could converse with, cajole, and possibly torture our younger siblings into agreeing with what we, the older sisters who obviously knew best, decided the "kids" wanted.

Twenty minutes later, returning to the living room, the four angels she was so proud of just a moment before announced to Mom that we had unanimously decided that we wanted to be in the movies! (Well, I announced it because it really was my idea. I'm the kid that was born to be a star.)

I can tell you she was surprised. "You're sure you don't want to go to Hawaii?"

"No, we want to be in the movies. Movies, movies," Bodie chanted.

That afternoon began yet another chapter in the lives of the Loy children. She did it. She gave us our reward. We had headshots taken by a professional photographer, and we signed up with an agent. For the next three years, Mom drove each of us down to LA as we were called to be extras. Our favorite job by far was the day we got paid to ride the roller coaster at Magic Mountain. After a few rides, one by one, the adult extras they had hired to make a Mylanta commercial started climbing out of the roller coaster. There they were, lying on the platform, holding their stomachs and moaning. Pretty soon it was just us four kids and Mom, riding the Colossus over and over. They shot the scene 33 times and then sent us over to the Revolution. I think we rode the Revolution about a dozen times. What a great day!

Mary and I stopped doing extra work when we got into high school. Spike and Bo held out until their acting careers threatened to interfere with baseball practice.

# 911—ONE, TWO, THREE, BOOM! YOU'RE GONE

After Spike had been away at college for a few months, he got really sick with the flu and his roommate had to call 911. This is the first time a super low blood sugar has ever happened to either of us. We put this in our book because maybe by understanding what happened to Spike, you can avoid ever getting this low. And don't get scared, everything turned out all right! Here is his e-mail.

Subj: low
Date: 2/5/99 9:24:48 a.m. Pacific Standard Time
From: Spike@stanford.edu
To: Bo

Had a rough day of snowboarding in some butt cold weather. Ate at Kentucky Fried Chicken on the way home. I ate a lot and took only 2/3 of my normal dose of insulin. The drive home from Tahoe was uneventful.

Then I get home and start feeling a little queasy and/or low. I test my blood sugar and I am about 70 [that's just the slightest bit low]. So I decide I had better eat a little to bring my sugar back up. I eat, but soon after I throw up quite a bit. This has happened before and I know that after throwing up I need to eat to replenish my sugars, so I eat and drink some more. I throw up a bunch again. I am feeling pretty bad at this point, pretty sick, and a little low, and really tired. I eat some more and lie down on my bed.

I wake up two hours later with five paramedics in my room, the residential fellow, two residential advisors and about four of my friends. But the cool stuff happened when I was unconscious and coming to.

Brad, my roommate, tells me that while lying in bed, I made a kind of gurgled mutter and fell out of bed (luckily I had just lowered my bed the week before). He kicked me or did something to try to rouse me, but I would have none of it, so he went and got Danny (our friend in the room across the hall). Danny couldn't wake me up and neither could Luke. So they called 911. The paramedics got there in two minutes flat (pretty good response time if you ask me—pretty reassuring).

Meanwhile, inside my head it felt like I was spinning. Each second or so I would see a new person in my room who was doing something new to me. The rate at which the strangers were flashing on the scene and bugging me started accelerating. I was spinning faster and faster, seeing someone new more and more rapidly and becoming more and more annoyed. Pretty psychedelic.

I remember thinking to myself, OK, Spike, this is just some dream. To make all these guys go away, so I can get some sleep, I just need to block them all out at once. I tried blocking them out. That didn't work. OK, then, I said to myself, I need to make them go away one by one.

I stood up, stared at one of the people in my room and said, "One, two, three, Boom! You're gone!" Then I looked through someone else and said, "One, two, three, Boom! You're gone!" After one, two, three, booming them away for a little while, the

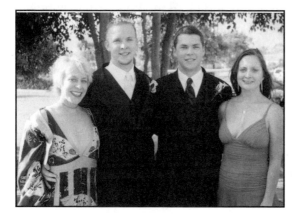

Jen, Bo, Spike,
and Mary—
all dressed up.

paramedics made me sit down, and shot me up with some glucagon. (That's an insulin inhibitor that gets the sugar to the brain faster.)

"Spike, can you hear me?"

"Who are you?"

"I'm Chris. I'm a paramedic. Can you hear me?"

"Yes."

"What day is it?"

"Ummm, Sunday night or Monday morning."

"Sure is."

I let out a sigh of relief. "Give me three seconds." I closed my eyes and counted, "One, two, three." I didn't say "Boom! You're gone" this time; I just opened my eyes and said, "Wow! You're still here."

"Spike, can you tell me who your friends are?"

"Sure." I looked around. "There's Luke. Brad's here, and Danny of course. Damn!"

The paramedics asked if I wanted to be hospitalized, and at first I said, yes, but pretty soon I was fully back to normal (as normal as I am ever gonna get) and I told them I was fine (which I was). I asked Chris what my sugar was, and he told me that when they first got there it was 39 [pretty low] but that it had risen to 370 or so [pretty high].

The paramedics all left, and my friends stuck around and made fun of me for a while, each one in turn imitating my "One, two, three, Boom! You're gone" routine. What good friends I've met here. Not only do they save my life, but they stick around to laugh about it. Golly.

**Note:** I had a second episode of falling blood sugars and the flu in February 2001. I called home for support and gave myself a glucagon injection. (My roommate could have done it, but I wanted to.) Within minutes my sugar was up and the low blood sugar episode passed. Don't be scared if you have to use glucagon. It works, and it won't hurt you.

Looking back on this incident, we know it happened because of a combination of things:

1. Spike took too much insulin. He had been exercising all day. He took ten units of Regular (short-acting) insulin at dinner, not his usual 15, but that was still too much. He should have taken only five or six units, even less.
2. He threw up. Remember the section, When You Are Sick, on page 115? Vomiting calls for special action. Throw up once: call someone. Throw up twice: get help.
3. His friends didn't know about glucagon. They do now! They did the right thing by calling 911, but they could have tried injecting Spike with glucagon when he wouldn't wake up. That would probably have been all that he needed.

We have written up a protocol for when you are sick: It's taped on Spike's closet door right now (see page 158). You may want to hang one like it up on yours, too.

## PROTOCOL FOR WHEN SPIKE IS SICK

* **Throw up once:** Tell a friend. Don't be alone. Call home so that they can check on you for the next few hours.
* **Throw up twice:** Go to the clinic at school. Don't go alone.
* **Glucagon:** Have your glucagon kit in your fridge. Tape the glucagon instructions on your closet door.
* **911:** Go ahead and call 911 if things get out of hand.

### Glucagon Instructions

**When Do You Use Glucagon?**

Inject Spike with glucagon if you can't wake him up or if he is so disoriented he doesn't make sense and you can't get him to eat.

**How Do You Use Glucagon?**

1. Inject the liquid in the syringe into the bottle of glucagon powder.
2. Shake the bottle until the glucagon dissolves and becomes clear.
3. Draw all the glucagon solution into the syringe. (For kids who weigh less than 45 pounds use half of the solution.)
4. Inject all the solution into Spike's leg or butt.
5. Put Spike on his side, because he may throw up when he wakes up.
6. Give him food as soon as he wakes up: Gatorade, crackers, cookies, or anything he can eat.

# 21 Tips

## Blood Sugar Testing

Don't prick the tips of your fingers; prick the sides of the finger pad—it feels better. With some new meters, you can prick your forearm. Be sure to rub your arm before pricking, so you'll get enough blood. Bo says it doesn't hurt.

## Cooler

Always have a packed cooler in any car you ride in. If you forget it, go back for it.

## Food

Keep a few dollars with you at all times in case you need to buy food.

At restaurants, order your food first. When it reaches the table, then take your insulin.

## Glucagon

Take a glucagon kit when you are traveling, camping, or backpacking.

## Hospitals

If you are going to the hospital, for example for surgery, take your kit and your cooler!

## Insulin and Injections

Throw away opened insulin after six weeks because it loses its potency.

For more comfortable injections, try an Inject-Ease. We found that it makes life easier. (An Inject-Ease is a device that puts the needle into the skin so you don't have to.)

Our favorite place to inject is the top of the hip. Sometimes we do it in the arm or the leg.

## Low Blood Sugar

When you have a low blood sugar, eat first and then test.

Always carry a granola bar in your pocket in case you get low.

We carry Cake Mate decorating gel—the $1.39 tube. It works when we're low.

For water sports, put a Cake Mate frosting in your wetsuit.

## Safety

Tell everyone you know that you have diabetes. You need to do this so that friends and grown-ups can help you when you are low and so that they can get involved.

When you go to school, go surfing, go to practice, go to a friend's, go in a car, or go anywhere, carry your backpack or a cooler. Then you are safe, and no one has to worry.

Wear a medical alert ID.

## Supplies

Have two of everything at home—insulin, fingerprick devices, batteries, Inject-Ease. Pumpers should have a second inserter at home, plus a supply of infusions sites and reservoirs. Things break.

Spike and I keep our syringes in five-gallon water bottles. When we are done with the syringes, we put the orange top back on but not the bottom white part because that makes it look like an unused syringe. Pharmacies also carry Sharps containers that you can use. At a friend's house, you can put the orange top back on your used syringes and then put them in an empty soda bottle or just keep them in your kit to take back home.

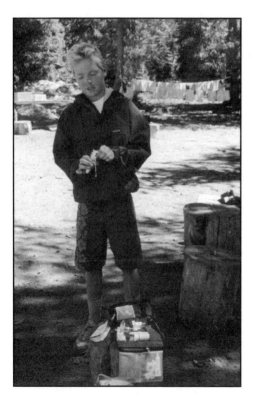

**Bo with his insulin kit while camping in Yosemite National Park, California.**

## Traveling

Take two sets of insulin on trips. Sometimes the glass bottles break. Keep insulin with you. It can freeze in the luggage compartment or go bad when it gets too hot. Take an extra battery for your glucose meter. If you are pumping, take extra pump batteries.

When we travel, we each carry backpacks containing our insulin kit, record book, Gatorade, frosting, crackers, cookies, and jerky. Have your mom or dad carry a back-up backpack, packed with the same things. Pumpers, have mom or dad carry back-up pump supplies.

# 22 Diabetes Research

We cannot stress enough how beneficial getting involved with research is. It gives us a great sense of hope. It also leads to a much greater understanding of what is going on with your condition. We have an ongoing scrapbook of our involvement, and it won't be finished until we can add the hospital papers documenting our successful islet cell transplants or the receipt from a closed loop continuous monitor and pump system.

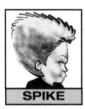

SPIKE

We met Dr. Patrick Soon-Shiong at the UCLA Transplant Lab in 1987. He told us how difficult it was to find pigs for research and asked for our help. Since we live on a small ranch, we were able to raise a special breed of pigs, Great Whites, for research. Great Whites have pancreatic cells that may someday be transplanted into humans. We raised them and slaughtered them, and my mother surgically removed their pancreases and transported them to Dr. Soon-Shiong's lab. Bo was six and I was eight when we started doing this, so our job was to be the timers. We timed how long it took to remove the pancreas and get it safely into the preservation solution. Bo sometimes actually put on surgical gloves and helped with the pancreas removal. We didn't have huge amounts of money to donate, but we did have space to raise these animals and time to do the weekly surgeries, so we did it. (We shared the meat with neighbors, so nothing was wasted.)

Being actively involved with the research gives me more hope for the future than anything else, and it has sparked my interest in entering the field of diabetes research as a profession after college.

## GET EXCITED ABOUT RESEARCH

Since we were diagnosed with diabetes, our family has been actively involved in diabetes research. There are currently many fields of research, ranging from looking for the cure to investigating technologies to make our lives even easier and to make diabetes even less of a nuisance. Here are some of the major fields of research.

### Stem Cell Research

On November 2, 2004, Californians voted overwhelming in favor of Proposition 71, the Stem Cell Research and Cures Initiative. Passage of this proposition established the California Institute of Regenerative Medicine (CIRM), whose charter is to make grants and provide loans for stem cell research, research facilities, and other vital research opportunities to the tune of $300 million a year for ten years. That's three billion dollars for stem cell research!

Although a lot of research needs to be done before stem cells can be used to treat kids with diabetes, it is a very exciting field these days. Stem cells have the potential to turn into all types of cells in your body: skin cells, blood cells, and, most important for us, islet cells, the cells that make insulin. The hope is that scientists can figure out how to get these stem cells to develop into fully functioning islet cells that can be implanted back into our bod-

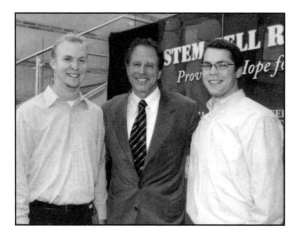

**Bo, Robert N. Klein, and Spike at a stem cell research rally.**

ies. It will be a while before scientists get this far, but it definitely seems like a possibility. Type 1 diabetes is high on the list of the conditions with the best chance of being treated with the therapies coming out of CIRM's work.

There are hurdles, though, both in the lab and in the courtroom. Scientists have to figure out how to keep our white blood cells from attacking new islet cells. (That's why we have diabetes to begin with; our white blood cells attacked our original insulin-making islet cells.) If they can solve that problem and if CIRM-funded and other researchers can figure out how to mass-produce islet cells, diabetes may someday be a thing of the past. With hard work and some lucky breakthroughs, our kids may just read about diabetes in history books.

Other hurdles involve the courts. Stem cell research is a touchy, sensitive subject in America. Some people think that using stem cells for science is wrong. They have their reasons, and they see their reasons as more important than our reasons for wanting stem cell research to go forward. The people who don't want this research to go on are taking the CIRM to court and holding up its work. I had an opportunity to hear some of their arguments in court, and I'm happy to say that it looks like the CIRM and stem cell research are going to win. Unfortunately, these lawsuits may keep the CIRM from getting to work for a couple of years.

Luckily, individuals and institutions have donated a lot of money to the CIRM, and in April 2006 the first grants were awarded to universities across the state of California. At that time, $14 million went out to train new stem cell scientists, who may be the ones to help cure diabetes. In the meantime, there are some things we can all do to help:

Stem cell research is touchy—you probably know plenty of good people on both sides of the debate. Talk to your family about where they stand on the issue.

If you are for stem cell research, write a letter to the elected officials in your state and let them know that you want your state to do research, too, just as California is doing.

Until the scientists make the big breakthroughs, researchers will have to get stem cells the old fashioned way—from people who donate their organs to science so that, after they are no longer living, other people can use their organs and islet cells to have better lives. Talk to your friends about becoming organ donors someday.

## Islet Transplants

This area of research involves transplanting human or pig islet cells into a person with diabetes. The islet cells are encapsulated in a semi-permeable membrane to protect them from the immune system. A successful transplant would eliminate the need for daily injections. (This is the field we were working on with Dr. Soon-Shiong.)

## Glucose Monitoring

Bo worked on a glucose-monitoring project when he did a summer internship at Medtronic MiniMed. The CGMS (continuous

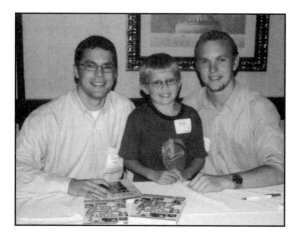

**Spike, Kyle, and Bo at a JDRF annual meeting.**

glucose-monitoring system) has a cannula like the one on the pump that delivers insulin, except that the CGMS cannula is fitted with a tiny sensor that monitors your blood sugars.

### The GlucoWatch Biographer
This research involves noninvasive glucose monitoring.

### Genetic Engineering
Genetic engineering research aims to create better forms of human insulin.

### Insulin Delivery Systems
Research is under way on developing better and smarter insulin pumps to replace daily injections. Nasal sprays and pills and insulin you can inhale are either in the works or just becoming available.

### Genetic Screening and Research
Screening of high-risk individuals who have a family history of diabetes and finding ways to prevent the immune system from destroying islet cells are two areas of genetic research that sci-

entists are currently investigating. A diabetes vaccine is also being studied.

Hundreds of labs are investigating diabetes around the country and around the globe. Donating money, time, or resources makes you feel like you are actually a part of the quest for the cure that is so close. Wouldn't it be great to be able to say, "I was a part of this" on the day that you get your cure?

# 23 Resources

Here is a list of our favorite diabetes products and supplies, along with some helpful books that you might want to read.

## THE SHOPPING LIST—
## OUR FAVORITE PRODUCTS
## AND SUPPLIES

### A1C Monitor

**Metrika A1C Now.** This is a great home-use monitor. This one-use, pager-sized device costs about $25 (you'll need a prescription) and gives you an A1C reading in minutes, with only a normal-sized drop of blood from a finger prick. Getting an A1C reading is important, because it gives you your blood sugar average for 3 months, which is necessary for good control. For example, if you had super high blood sugars at night that you weren't catching with your normal testing regimen, your A1C average would be high and alert you to the problem. We used to dread getting our A1Cs done, because it meant a costly trip to the lab and blood had to be drawn from our veins.

## Cooler

**Playmate Little Igloo.** Available at sporting goods stores for about $15.00. We keep a packed cooler in each car—even our girl-friends' cars. At college, we still carry a cooler everywhere.

## Frosting (Tube)

**Cake Mate decorating gel** (net weight 0.68 oz/19 g). Available in all grocery stores. Each small tube contains 45 calories and costs $1.39. We buy them by the dozen and have them all over the house—in backpacks, coolers, our kits, and the glove compartments of cars. They are so cheap that you can put them everywhere, including up the sleeve of a wet suit. We like the white cake frosting.

## Frosting (Tub)

We always keep a tub of **Duncan Hines Home Style Creamy Frosting** (**Chocolate Malt**) in the cupboard. If you keep it in the cupboard, then it's soft when you need to use it. We use it on graham crackers when we are low and by the tablespoon when we are very low. We take it on camping trips.

## Gels (Sports)

**Power Bar Power Gel** (28 g carb per pack) and **Gu** (28 g carb per pack w/caffeine). These work fast and taste pretty good! They cost $1.00–$2.50 each. Runners and bicycle riders like Lance Armstrong use it. Found in bicycle and running shops.

## Glucagon Kit

Always keep a **Glucagon Kit** on hand. Take it when you travel. It works like magic for very low blood sugar. It stops the action of insulin and raises blood sugar. You'll need a prescription. A kit costs about $90.

## Glucose Tabs and Glucose Gel

Glucose tabs are used for relieving low blood sugar. Each tab contains 4 or 5 grams of carbohydrate. Read the label. Glucose gel is used for treating low blood sugar. Each tube contains 24 grams of carbohydrate. (We keep candy bars and other sugary foods around to eat when we are low. We figure that if you are going to be low and you have to eat sugar, it might as well be something you like.) Available at pharmacies.

## Ice Packs

The Refrigerant Gel Pack that comes with Medicool's Dia-Pak (see Insulin Kit, below) lasts about a week. You will need to buy three small (3 inch by 5 inch) hard plastic ice packs. Microban also makes an ice pack called Lunch-Pak. They are available in sporting goods stores.

## Injection Device

**Inject-Ease (Palco Labs).** This device made it a lot easier to give ourselves our first shots. You drop the syringe into the rocket-ship-looking Inject-Ease and press a button. The device sends the needle into you fast. Then you push the plunger down to deliver the insulin. Available at pharmacies.

## Insulin Kit

**Medicool's Dia-Pak.** It's big enough to hold a week's worth of syringes, three bottles of insulin, a granola bar, frosting, our meter kit, and more if need be. Order the Dia-Pak Diabetic Supply Organizer by Medicool at 1-800-433-2469. The address is Medicool, 23520 Telo Ave., Suite #6, Torrance, CA 90505. The cost of carrying kits ranges from $15.95 for the simplest daypack to $29.95 for the deluxe model. Medicool is featured in the "Shopper's Guide" portion of the ADA's publication *Diabetes Forecast.*

### Insulin Vial Protector

**Insure Insulin Vial Protector 2,** available through Medport. Individual vial holders cost $4.95 each. Good for travel and backpacking. Go to www.medportinc.com to order.

### Ketostix

**Reagent Strips for Urinalysis by Bayer.** They are available at just about any pharmacy. We buy the simple ketone test strips. Some strips also show a color for blood sugar, but you are already doing blood sugar with your arm or finger prick test. There's less information to digest when you check for ketones if you use the simple ketone-only strip. A bottle of 50 costs about $12.95.

### Lancet Devices (Pricker)

**TheraSense FreeStyle.** It works on the arm, and it's awesome. TheraSense introduced us to the idea of testing our forearms or legs, and we like the testing device they provide. Testing the forearm is painless, and you have a much larger surface area to work with.

**BD Lancet Device.** If you are still testing your blood via the fingertips, we like the BD Lancet device. They last a long time, and you can adjust them for depth if you're having trouble getting blood out of your finger. They cost about $12.95.

### Lancets

**BD Ultra Fine II.** These lancets seem to be a little slimmer and they feel better than others. They work with the TheraSense lancet device. A box of 200 costs $15–$17.

## MedicAlert

**MedicAlert Bracelet or Necklace.** Available for $35. Contact MedicAlert at 1-800-432-5378 or Medical ID jewelry at www.laurenshope.com.

## Meters

**OneTouch Ultra (LifeScan).** We really like this meter. It is super-small, uses only a tiny bit of blood, and gives you a reading in just 5 seconds! If you like testing your forearm instead of your fingers, you can use a OneTouch Ultra for that, too. Visit www.lifescan.com or call 1-800-227-8862 for more information. This meter costs about $70 (but pharmacies sometimes have promotions where they give the meter away when you buy 100 strips). The cost of 100 strips is about $75.

**OneTouch UltraSmart (LifeScan).** This new meter has loads of tracking and trending capabilities (like the TheraSense Tracker, below) and gives results in just 5 seconds, like the OneTouch Ultra.

**TheraSense Tracker.** We just got two of these, and they are great. You can keep track of all your information easily and see trends to help you get a better grip on your diabetes. The cost of the PDS (Personal Digital System), module, and software is about $299, but it comes with a $75 rebate. Module and software only are $149, with a $40 rebate (you would then use your own PDA, such as a HandSpring or Visor).

**TheraSense Freestyle.** If the Tracker costs more than you want to spend, or you just don't feel like storing all that information all the time, we still recommend the TheraSense meter. Bo uses it and loves it. It uses very little blood, and you can take up to a minute and a half to get blood on the strip. The FreeStyle is available from www.therasense.com or 1-888-522-5226. (Some drugstores have specials where you get the meter free if you buy a bottle of strips.) The cost of meter is $75, and it comes with a $40 mail-in rebate. The cost of 100 strips is $69.95.

## Snack Bars

**Extend Bar.** Good before-bed snack. Helps stabilize blood sugar for up to 9 hours. Go to www.extendbarworks.com. Four bars cost about $5.00.

**Glucerna Bar.** Tasty snack bars. Use them when playing sports. Get them at www.glucerna.com. Four bars cost about $6.50.

**NiteBite Bar.** Made with cornstarch. They help keep blood sugars level during the night. Good before-bed snack.

**PowerBars and Clif Bars.** These are packed with carbs. Lots of kids eat them when they are into heavy exercise!

## Sugar-Free Cookies

We discovered **Murray Sugar-Free Shortbread and Sandwich Cookies** at the 2002 ADA Convention in San Francisco. Tasty.

## Syringes

When Bo and Spike used syringes, Bo used **BD Ultra Fine II** and Spike used the **BD Ultra Fine II Short Needle**. Bo used an injection device. He found that using the device with the short needle didn't get the needle in deep enough and hurt sometimes. Spike just injected by hand, so he preferred the shorter needle.

# OTHER BOOKS TO READ

If you would like to learn more about diabetes, here are books we recommend. All are available at bookstores, Amazon.com, and store.diabetes.org. (Contact us at *spikeandbo@gmail.com*.)

*487 Really Cool Tips for Kids with Diabetes,* by us and about 114 other kids.

*Real Life Parenting of Kids with Diabetes,* by Virginia Nasmyth Loy. This companion book to *Getting a Grip* is the how-to book for parents, teachers, coaches, and friends. *Real Life Parenting* includes a large section on toddlers and a chapter on going off to college.

*Cooking Up Fun for Kids with Diabetes,* by Patti B. Geil, MS, RD, CDE, and Tami A. Ross, RD, CDE. Have fun creating cool and diabetes-friendly kids' foods.

*The Diabetes Travel Guide, 2nd edition,* by Davida Kruger. This handy book helps you organize traveling with diabetes.

*A Field Guide to Type 1 Diabetes,* by ADA. A good exploration of diabetes and how to live with it.

*Getting the Most Out of Diabetes Camp: A Guidebook for Parents and Kids,* by ADA.

*An Instructional Aid on Juvenile Diabetes Mellitus,* by Luther B. Travis, MD.

*Smart Pumping for People with Diabetes,* by Howard Wolpert, MD. Everything you'll need to know about insulin pumps by a Joslin Center pump master.

*Taking Diabetes to School,* by Kim Grossalin et al. This is a good book for grade-school kids to share with their teachers and fellow students.

# Index

athletics, 34, 44–46, 93. *See also* sports

attitude about diabetes, 147–152

## B

backpacking, 41–43, 75–83

basal rate, 8, 91, 93

baseline, 91, 93

beer, 67–70, 115

beta cells, 2

bicycling, 38–40

blood cells, 2–3

blood circulation, 68

blood sugar control, 91, 93–94, 107, 109, 111.
　　*See also* hyperglycemia; hypoglycemia

blood sugar, high. *See* hyperglycemia

blood sugar, low. *See* hypoglycemia

blood testing, 163, 166, 169, 172

bolus, 91, 93, 111

brain, 6

brothers, 147–153

bubble shields, 3

## C

California Institute of Regenerative Medicine, xvi, 164–166

calories, 116–118

camp, 25–30

Camp Conrad Chinnock, 27–30

energy, lack of, 4, 8. *See also* hyperglycemia; hypoglycemia

epinephrine, 113

excursions, 25–30

exercise, 34, 44–46, 93. *See also* sports

exhaustion, 44–45

## F

fainting, 5–6, 140. *See also* hypoglycemia

family, 147–153

fatigue, 6. *See also* hypoglycemia

*Field Guide to Type 1 Diabetes* (ADA), 175

flu, 115. *See also* hyperglycemia; hypoglycemia; illness; ketones

food

    calories, 116–118

    carbohydrate, 6, 14–17, 33–34, 125–137

    categories, 125–127

    "cheating", 108–109

    driving, and, 64–65

    excursions, and, 26–27

    illness, and, 112

    menu, 130–133

    proteins, 135–137

    recommendations, 170, 174

    restaurants, 51–53

    school, and, 47–48, 72

    sports, and, 32–43

    travel, and, 56–58

food poisoning, 115–118. *See also* hyperglycemia; hypoglycemia; illness; ketones forms, 139, 142–145

*487 Really Cool Tips for Kids with Diabete*s, 89, 126, 175

Freestyle Tracker, 12–13. *See also* glucose monitor

Fulkerson, Tracy, 29


## G

Geil, Patti B., *Cooking Up Fun for Kids with Diabetes*, 175

genetic engineering, 167

genetic screening, 167–168

*Getting the Most Out of Diabetes Camp* (ADA), 175

glucagon (hormone), 6, 113, 119–120

glucagon kit(s), 19, 38, 42, 57, 86, 170

glucose, 1, 6, 171

glucose monitor, 163, 166–167, 169, 173

GlucoWatch Biographer, 167

Great White pigs, 163–164

Grossalin, Kim, *Taking Diabetes to School*, 176

growth hormone, 113

growth spurt, 8, 145


## H

headache, 4, 6, 140. *See also* hyperglycemia; hypoglycemia

heart attack, 69

hormones
    adrenaline, 6
    cortisol, 113
    epinephrine, 113

# I

## J

JDRF (Juvenile Diabetes Research Foundation), 23, 167

jellyfish, 61

Juvenile Diabetes Research Foundation, 23, 167

## K

ketoacidosis, 118

ketones, 7, 9, 111, 113–118, 172

Kids with Diabetes Inc., 23

kit(s), 11–19, 42, 55–61, 64, 92–93, 171.
    *See also* diabetes, supplies

Kruger, Davida, *Diabetes Travel Guide*, 175

## L

languages, foreign, 80–83

light-headedness, 6. *See also* hypoglycemia

Loy, Bo. xiii–xvii
    *487 Really Cool Tips for Kids with Diabetes,* 89, 126, 175

Loy, Jenny, 151–153

Loy, Mary, "Why Animals Are Used In Biomedical
    Research," 148–151

Loy, Spike. xiii–xvii
    *487 Really Cool Tips for Kids with Diabetes,* 89, 126, 175

Loy, Virginia, *Real Life Parenting of Kids with
    Diabetes,* 73, 175

## M

marijuana, 69–70

medical I.D., 57, 61, 64–65, 160, 173

MedicAlert, 173

medications, 16, 59–61, 112

Medicool Dia-Pak, 13, 171

Medtronic MiniMed, 97, 103–104

mellitus. *See* diabetes

menu, 130–133

meter kit(s), 12–14, 18

meter, testing, 163, 166–167, 169, 173

Metrika A1C Now, 169

motorcycling, 38–41

muscles, 44–45

## N

narcotics, 67–70

Nasmyth Loy, Bo, *See* Loy, Bo

Nasmyth Loy, Spike, *See* Loy, Spike

Nasmyth Loy, Virginia, *See* Loy, Virginia

nausea, 111–112. *See also* hyperglycemia;
  ketoacidosis

## O

Ojai Kids, 23

organ transplant, 2–3, 109, 163–168

organs, *see under* individual organs

Outdoor School, 25–30

outings, 25–30

## P

PADRE Foundation, 23

palpitations, 6. *See also* hypoglycemia

pancreas, 1–3, 109

parents, 147–153

partying, 67–70

Permission to Treat form, 139

pharmacies, 56, 80

physical fitness, 34, 44–46, 93. *See also* sports

physicians, 107–109

pigs, Great White, 163–164

Playmate Little Igloo, 170

Proposition 71, 164–166

proteins, 135–137

pump, 89–105, 114, 163, 167. *See also* diabetes, supplies; kit(s)

## R

*Real Life Parenting of Kids with Diabetes* (Nasmyth Loy, Virginia), 73, 175

research, 148–151, 163–168

restaurants, 51–53

# S

sugar, 1, 3

supplies, 11–19, 55–61, 77–80, 83, 161, 169–174

support groups, 21, 23–24

surfing, 35–38

surgery, 121–123

sweating, 6. *See also* hypoglycemia

symptoms

    anger, 140

    clammy, 8

    consciousness, loss of, 5–6, 140

    convulsions, 5–6

    crying, 5, 140

    depression, 3

    diabetes, 1

    drowsiness, 6

    energy, lack of, 4, 8

    fainting, 5–6, 140

    fatigue, 6

    headache, 4, 6, 140

    hunger, 6, 140

    hyperglycemia. *See* hyperglycemia

    hypoglycemia. *See* hypoglycemia

    irritability, 5–6, 140

    light-headedness, 6

    palpitations, 6

    shakiness, 4, 6, 140

    stomachache, 4, 140

    sweating, 6

    thirst, 7

    unresponsive, 5

    urination, frequent, 7

# T

# U

# V

# W

water, effect of cold on blood sugars, 27, 35

Weigensberg, Marc J. Dr., xvii

white blood cells, 2–3

"Why Animals Are Used In Biomedical Research"
   (Loy, Mary), 148–151

Wilson, Rocky Dr., 30

Wolpert, Howard, *Smart Pumping for People with Diabetes,* 176

# Other Titles Available from the American Diabetes Association

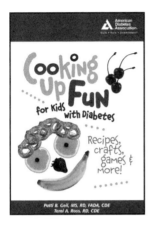

## Cooking Up Fun for Kids with Diabetes

*By Patti Geil, MS, RD, FADA, CDE, and Tami Ross, RD, LD, CDE*

This fun-filled book is the perfect way to banish boredom in the kitchen forever. Packed with simple, healthy recipes, projects, and activities, *Cooking Up Fun for Kids with Diabetes* is a great way to get the whole family involved in healthy eating.

Order #4641-01 • $14.95 US

## Guide to Healthy Restaurant Eating, 3rd Edition

*By Hope S. Warshaw, MMSc, RD, CDE, BC-ADM*

Eat out without guilt or sacrifice! Newly updated, this bestselling guide features more than 5,000 menu items for over 60 restaurant chains. This is the most comprehensive guide to restaurant nutrition for people with diabetes who like to eat out.

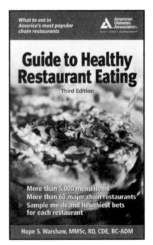

Order #4819-03 • $17.95 US

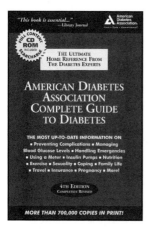

## American Diabetes Association Complete Guide to Diabetes, 4th Edition

*By the American Diabetes Association*
The world's largest collection of diabetes self-care tips, techniques, and tricks you can use to solve diabetes-related troubles just got bigger and better!
Order #4809-04 • $29.95 US

## 101 Tips for Raising Healthy Kids with Diabetes

*By Laura Hieronymus, MSEd, APRN, BC-ADM, CDE and Patti Geil, MS, RD, FADA, CDE*
Dealing with the unexpected twists and turns as a child with diabetes grows and develops can be overwhelming. That's why there's *101 Tips for Raising Healthy Kids with Diabetes.* A quick and easy read,

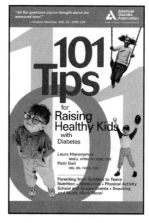

the Q&A format contains essential advice on everything from medication to nutrition to special situations.
Order #4920-01 • $14.95 US

**Order online at http://store.diabetes.org or call toll-free at 1-800-232-6733.**

# About the American Diabetes Association

The American Diabetes Association is the nation's leading voluntary health organization supporting diabetes research, information, and advocacy. Its mission is to prevent and cure diabetes and to improve the lives of all people affected by diabetes. The American Diabetes Association is the leading publisher of comprehensive diabetes information. Its huge library of practical and authoritative books for people with diabetes covers every aspect of self-care—cooking and nutrition, fitness, weight control, medications, complications, emotional issues, and general self-care.

To order American Diabetes Association books: Call 1-800-232-6733 or log on to *http://store.diabetes.org*

To join the American Diabetes Association: Call 1-800-806-7801 or log on to *www.diabetes.org/membership*

For more information about diabetes or ADA programs and services: Call 1-800-342-2383. E-mail: AskADA@diabetes.org or log on to *www.diabetes.org*

To locate an ADA/NCQA Recognized Provider of quality diabetes care in your area: *www.ncqa.org/dprp*

To find an ADA Recognized Education Program in your area: Call 1-800-342-2383. *www.diabetes.org/for-health-professionals-and-scientists/recognition/edrecognition.jsp*

To join the fight to increase funding for diabetes research, end discrimination, and improve insurance coverage: Call 1-800-342-2383. *www.diabetes.org/advocacy-and-legalresources/advocacy.jsp*

To find out how you can get involved with the programs in your community: Call 1-800-342-2383. See below for program Web addresses.

- American Diabetes Month: educational activities aimed at those diagnosed with diabetes—month of November. www.diabetes.org/communityprograms-and-localevents/americandiabetesmonth.jsp

- American Diabetes Alert: annual public awareness campaign to find the undiagnosed—held the fourth Tuesday in March. *www.diabetes.org/communityprograms-and-localevents/americandiabetesalert.jsp*

- American Diabetes Association Latino Initiative: diabetes awareness program targeted to the Latino community. *www.diabetes.org/communityprograms-and-localevents/latinos.jsp*

- African American Program: diabetes awareness program targeted to the African American community. *www.diabetes.org/communityprograms-and-localevents/africanamericans.jsp*

- Awakening the Spirit: Pathways to Diabetes Prevention & Control: diabetes awareness program targeted to the Native American community. *www.diabetes.org/communityprograms-and-localevents/nativeamericans.jsp*

To find out about an important research project regarding type 2 diabetes: *www.diabetes.org/diabetes-research/research-home.jsp*

To obtain information on making a planned gift or charitable bequest: Call 1-888-700-7029. *www.wpg.cc/stl/CDA/homepage/1,1006,509,00.html*

To make a donation or memorial contribution: Call 1-800-342-2383. *www.diabetes.org/support-the-cause/make-a-donation.jsp*